THE
SOBER
LUSH

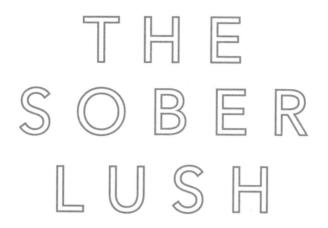

THE SOBER LUSH

A HEDONIST'S GUIDE TO LIVING A DECADENT,
ADVENTUROUS, SOULFUL LIFE—ALCOHOL FREE

AMANDA EYRE WARD
AND JARDINE LIBAIRE

A TarcherPerigee Book

tarcherperigee

an imprint of Penguin Random House LLC
penguinrandomhouse.com

A version of "Room 302" appeared in *Texas Monthly* as
"What's Going Down in Room 312" in February 2017.
A version of "Climbing Rocks" appeared in *Self* as
"Why a Little Risk Is Good for You" in 2015.

Most Tarcher/Penguin books are available at special quantity discounts for bulk purchase for sales promotions, premiums, fund-raising, and educational needs. Special books or book excerpts also can be created to fit specific needs. For details, write SpecialMarkets@penguinrandomhouse.com.

Library of Congress Cataloging-in-Publication Data

Names: Libaire, Jardine, author. | Ward, Amanda Eyre, 1972– author.
Title: The sober lush : a hedonist's guide to living a decadent, adventurous,
soulful life—alcohol free / Jardine Libaire and Amanda Eyre Ward.
Description: [New York] : TarcherPerigee, an imprint of Penguin Random House LLC, [2020]
Identifiers: LCCN 2020006475 (print) | LCCN 2020006476 (ebook) |
ISBN 9780593084823 (hardcover) | ISBN 9780593084830 (ebook)
Subjects: LCSH: Temperance. | Drinking of alcoholic beverages—Psychological aspects. |
Drinking of alcoholic beverages—Health aspects.
Classification: LCC HV5060 .L483 2020 (print) | LCC HV5060 (ebook) | DDC 613.81—dc23
LC record available at https://lccn.loc.gov/2020006475
LC ebook record available at https://lccn.loc.gov/2020006476
p.   cm.

Printed in the United States of America
1   3   5   7   9   10   8   6   4   2

Book design by Laura K. Corless

Amanda would like to dedicate this book to
the loved ones who inspired her path,
Gary Davenport Brabander Ward,
Larry and Barbara Meckel, Peter Westley,
and to her partner in crime, Jardine.

Jardine dedicates this book to all the Ravens,
who showed her how luscious life can be,
and to her dear ally Amanda.

CONTENTS

EATING

COPING

CONSCIOUSNESS EXPERIMENTS

PLAYING

IN YOUR GLASS

LOVE

TINY MAGIC CONNECTIONS

SLOWING DOWN

CREATING

ROAMING

LAGNIAPPE

INTRODUCTION

We are writers. We fell in love with the elegant, gin-soaked stories of Raymond Carver, Jean Rhys, Patricia Highsmith, Dorothy Parker, and Ernest Hemingway. We were seduced by the druggy prose of Hunter S. Thompson, Helen Garner, and Paul Bowles. We wrote our own short stories with a glass of whiskey next to our notebooks, tapping lipstick-stained cigarettes into an ashtray stolen from a hotel we could not afford.

We dreamed of being novelists and listened to Johnny Thunders and Billie Holiday and Jimi Hendrix and stayed too late in bars that were open past closing time and we woke with a pounding in our heads and our hearts. We wanted to make something true and beautiful, wanted a surefire way to get to the other side of ordinary life—to the creative side, the anarchistic side, the hedonistic side.

We hit a wall in this pursuit when drinking did not deliver us to that hallowed place of creating and dreaming and living big. Instead, it took us further away. We knew our lives needed to change, and so we searched for the answers in books. We found Pete Hamill's *A*

Drinking Life; Caroline Knapp's *Drinking, A Love Story*; Sarah Hepola's *Blackout*; and Mary Karr's *Lit*. We devoured the stories of artists who'd almost boozed themselves to death but then decided, instead, to live. These incredible books were the entry point into imagining something else, and their accounts of lost weekends, blacked-out days, and broken families helped us know it was time to stop. But we also wondered, *Is this the end, or can it be a beginning?*

We were introduced to each other because we were both sober writers, and when we sat down to talk, we had many of the same questions. Both of us had given up drinking in our own ways, through our own processes, but now wondered how to *thrive* sober.

We talked for hours, meeting in Jardine's garden or walking the trail around Austin's Lady Bird Lake. Amanda cried while Jardine's Chihuahua, Loverman, lay curled at her side, his eyes as beseeching as Amanda's voice. We went to meetings; we went to lunch. We drank coffee and more coffee.

What happens when you decide to live sober—for a month or a lifetime—but still yearn for danger and chaos, still hope for a secret path to joy? How can you find the sort of raw and crazy connection that used to come in boozy, dive-bar confession sessions? Can you still be dirty and wild, can you take a super-blissed-out vacation, can you trip out on life, can you fall in love, holding a *ginger ale*?

The *Oxford English Dictionary* defines *sober* as "abstaining from drinking" and also, problematically, as "somber, quiet, inward, responsible, humorless." But we have no interest in spending our lives being solemn, grave, staid, serious, logical! The fear that *this* was the nature of a sober life kept us from even considering it for years, long after our gut had told us to check out.

The idea of this book is to redefine lushness and reclaim it. For ourselves and many we know, figuring out sobriety has been lonely, and we don't think it needs to be, so this book is a way to keep one another company while we plot a new course. Our stories here are sometimes about alcohol, or the absence of it, but more often they're about orchids and ice cream and mountains and basil and shooting stars and roller skates and Ethiopian coffee and sex and vetiver and horses and masquerades and glitter. This is on purpose.

Once upon a time, we thought of sobriety as doing without, as giving up, as deprivation, as substitution. Now our philosophy is rooted in abundance and pleasure. We love seeing parallel approaches, like vegetarians who no longer make a turkey out of tofu but rather serve a feast of ripe tomatoes and garden zucchini and toasted pine nuts and sweet potato with a homemade tahini sauce and grilled halloumi and naan with a dessert of ginger sorbet and pomegranate. They have rethought culinary pleasure from the ground up. Or a friend who wanted to get strong but didn't *just* give up junk food and sugar—he started kickboxing and learned to cook exquisitely and bikes to work, and he's stronger but also more alive.

Sober lushness is not a moral code, and not a closed club. It's a loose set of ideas and experiences that anyone is welcome to use, and we're all free to come and go as we please. We don't believe in sides; we don't see it as sober people versus drinkers. We don't imagine someone as in or out.

For this reason, we decided to use the "we" voice to invite as many readers as possible to connect. Some of these stories belong to one of us and some are closer to being universal.

This book is not meant to prescribe a way of life, or to show that one way of living is better than another. This book is not against alcohol—we know many people who drink and drinking doesn't do to their lives what it did to ours. This book is simply a collection of the beautiful lovely things that we do (or dream of doing) that link us to the creative and rebellious side of being sober, now that we have given up drinking because—for personal and particular reasons—it was a good thing to do for ourselves.

We do not claim to know who else might want to go down that road; that choice is up to the individual. Part of what we believe— that actually led us to say *no thank you* to a drinking life in the first place—is that we like to live the way we want, and f*%k social pressure to live any other way.

The spectrum of human beings who play with sober hedonism is large and diverse, including women and men, old and young, from all backgrounds, famous and anonymous, newly sober or sage warriors lighting our path, and they do it for a spectrum of reasons too. Some of us are just starting to explore, some have been committed to sobriety for decades, some are curious about moderation, some have survived life-and-death crises with substances, but sober hedonism is a meeting place for anyone. No one is excluded.

We don't want to intimate that this book is full of answers and prescriptions and therapeutic advice. We are dreamers and storytellers who have made a hundred mistakes and have more questions than conclusions and who see life as a crazy journey and not a blueprint. So we offer our stories—since we love stories and the way they connect people, the way they can sometimes heal the teller and heal the listener, and bring light to darkness.

While this book will hopefully reach you, we do want to say that we understand—with all our hearts—that for many of us, a book— *any* book—is not nearly enough to get sober, or to stay sober. So this collection isn't meant to take the place of all the many resources out there that can help. This book isn't a detox program or a 12-step meeting or a counselor or a sponsor. We have personally found that connection to others is key to staying sober, and sober connections are available to all who seek them, online or in a room.

This is not a textbook as much as an offering. Feel free to use it as you would a swimming hole: dive deep or take a quicksilver dip.

And we hope that wherever you are in your precious life, you can take and leave what you need for your own plan. For example, some people in recovery are triggered by nonalcoholic cocktails to want to drink alcohol again; if you fear that might affect you, please skip the "In Your Glass" section and the last chapter of recipes, both of which discuss zero-proof drinks. We made the decision to include these chapters not to mimic our past habits but because we love to eat and sip delicious things. But that is how *we* feel. We have respect and love for the autonomy of each reader, the unique path of every human being, and hope you'll use the book as it suits you.

Welcome, reader, to a story that is not as much about what is lost but what is found. It's an idiosyncratic manual, from the heart. We begin with two pieces on how we each got to where we are now, then the chapters are loosely gathered around certain aspects of life, finishing with an array of recipes. But there is no order or regimen implied, no correct place to start or finish.

If you're wondering whether you're in the right spot, come sit on our tattered black velvet sofa and we'll pour you a ginger beer, offer you some angel cake, and put a record on the turntable. Take your time and decide for yourself.

Are you wondering if you might be happier tonight without a drink? Are you pregnant, seeking a new way into the fun? Have you been sober for ten years? Are you starting a dry January, or October—any month off sugar and booze? Are you curious about living a giant, dirty, wild, glamorous life without consequences of numbness or regret? Are you a parent who wants to be more present for your children? Do you occasionally google "Am I an alcoholic"? Are you in the middle of a fabulous career but feeling lost? Are you single and worried about dating sober? Are you in a relationship and a big part of the relationship is drinking? Are you lonely in having these questions or this uncertainty and you wonder if other people are wondering about all this? Are you in college, curious about the ways your life can unfold? Do you drink because you don't want to be a killjoy, even as you're asking yourself, *Where's the joy?* Are you scared that if you don't drink, you will be even more scared? Is there a small, true voice from somewhere inside you saying, *Do I want this to be my story?*

Welcome.

We wrote this book for you.

JADE EARRINGS

AMANDA'S STORY

When I woke, I was still in my New Year's Eve dress, my second son asleep next to me. My jade earrings were gone. I checked both bedside tables but found only books and a half-filled glass of Chardonnay. I had hosted a party the night before and could remember that the fireworks had been lit before midnight. After that, I remembered nothing.

My son's perfect face, awash in slumber. The Colorado sun, slanting in the window of the master bedroom, pale against the snow. I tried anxiously to determine where I'd left my earrings. They were large and flashy—jubilant. They'd been a Christmas present to myself.

I slipped on my robe over silver velvet, tying the sash tight. My hair still smelled of the fancy hairstyle I'd made stick with Aqua Net as I prepared for the party, sipping wine from a large goblet. One of my black heels lay next to the bed. I felt a sour panic as I scanned the room for the other, but ah, there it was, by the doorway.

I went to check on my toddler daughter, who was curled up and breathing softly. I found my eldest son sprawled on his top bunk wearing snow pants. My heart slowed, knowing all three were safe, but the dread would remain for days.

I'd googled the dread many times—was it chemical, something about the Chardonnay going sludgy in my veins? Was I an alcoholic? Did I need to stop drinking forever? (I want to tell myself, my poor, desperate teenage/college-age/middle-aged self, if you google these questions, then yes. Just yes. You don't have to be done, but my God, you are allowed to be.)

I was nine when I told my father (after taking a quiz on the back of an AA pamphlet) that he was an alcoholic. I remember standing next to the cupboard where he kept his handles of Jack Daniel's. My two younger sisters and I were terrified of him: I never knew when he'd scream at us for running up the goddamn stairs, slam my shoulders to the ground and ask me how it felt to be a failure, or chastise us for being spoiled rotten. There is a small child who lives inside me that is so scared of him, even now, that I feel sick and sometimes tremble when I think of those days. I don't remember many of them at all.

My earrings were not in the kitchen, where I made coffee and took four New Year's Day Advil. I took Benadryl every night, too, to shut down my brain and sleep, though I had no idea if I'd done so the night before.

After a blackout, I was a miserable detective searching for clues. What had I done? Would an earring be found under the bed of a man on the other side of town? Had I said something to my husband for which he would never forgive me?

On one of my last drinking nights, I insisted on a "double Chardonnay to go" from the bartender. Someone posted a photograph of me on Facebook, holding a large solo cup, laughing. I don't remember the photo. I don't remember ordering a double Chardonnay. It's me in the picture, but it's not me. Who is it?

To others, I seemed absolutely fine. I drank normally for months at a time, enjoying a glass or two of wine in the evenings or even not drinking at all . . . but try as I might, I couldn't keep from eventually overdoing it. I later met sober friends who talked about trying—as I had—to find the "third door," when you don't want to quit, but you can't seem to moderate. A new life opened when I finally accepted that, for me, there is no third door.

My daughter appeared on New Year's Day, her arms embracing my leg. "You're OK," I told my daughter.

She looked up at me quizzically. She said, "Mama, can we read books now?"

I filled a mug with hot coffee and sat in the front room. My daughter nestled in, her thumb in her mouth, her cheek next to my robe's ivory-colored fake fur. As I opened *Madeleine* and read, my son and then my other son woke and came toward me. Here I was: the mother I wanted, so very much, to be.

I promised myself I would never—absolutely never, no matter what—drink more than four glasses of wine in one night again.

By February, I would make this promise a lie.

Even as I type this, I want a glass of Chardonnay.

I have never found my jade earrings.

When I was fifteen, my father got sober. In the end, his struggle became the greatest gift he could ever give me: the understanding of how alcohol could wreck your heart, and the living example that you could burn your way to freedom.

On my eldest son's fifteenth birthday, I had given up the search for the third door; I'd been sober for two years. After a celebratory family dinner, I settled into bed with a book. Around 8:00 p.m., my son appeared in the doorway. He wore shorts and a T-shirt. "Hey, Mom," he said.

I looked up.

"I'm going on a quick run. Want to come?"

I had once been the kind of mom who said, "I'm already in my pajamas." I used to be three glasses deep into a bottle of Chardonnay by 8:00 p.m. But I closed my book, losing my place. I threw back the sheets. I said, "Why not?"

The sun was low in the sky. A rainstorm had just come through, and it was cool, the night smelling of asphalt and magnolia. My son, a cross-country runner, was fast. "Go on ahead," I said. He nodded and picked up his pace.

I watched him go, fifteen years after I'd first held him in my arms. I slowed to a walk, then stood still, overwhelmed by a thundering, simple peace. My son would run to the end of the road, turn around, and come back. I would be there, my cheeks hot and my eyes filled with tears. He'd smile when he saw his mother.

All the fear of the first sober months, the exhaustion of searching for another way to be, the confusion of finding a new tribe in the middle of a life, the nights I wanted just one sip or a whole bottle of Chardonnay. The cans and cans of seltzer. Tears on Jardine's couch.

The moon emerged overhead and I knew: it was for this.

THE FURIOUS TURQUOISE

JARDINE'S STORY

August on Long Island, and I'm seven and standing with my family on the dock; we're stepping one by one onto our boat to head over to Fire Island, to anchor with other boats, all friends of ours, all families, and spend this Sunday swimming, eating ham sandwiches, hunting for beach glass. There's haze and brine in the low sky today. The moms—in giant 1970s sunglasses—light cigarettes and talk as they sunbathe in the cockpits of the boats. The fathers are cowboys, hip-deep in the gray dazzle of the bay, holding beers aloft.

After lunch, we all walk across the narrow island to the ocean side, where we kids spend hours riding the surf, high on the crest of a wave, falling, getting tumbled, rising again. As the sun sets, milky and pink, we putter home—everyone alone with their thoughts, tired but together—in the potbellied old boat. On the shore, an egret primly picks her way through seaweed and driftwood toward dusk. That night, I close my eyes to sleep and all I see is the endless cycle of turquoise water, the beautiful and terrifying surf—because

I'd been consumed by the ocean that day, part of something bigger than my tiny self, and so alive.

Now I'm fifteen, and my weirdo misfit friends and I find a treehouse in the woods, and we climb up to hang out there in the blue autumn afternoon, smoking Camel Lights and filling out notebooks together, leaves blazing magenta and yellow around us. We don't drink yet, we don't do drugs, we just write poems and lists of absurd things, and we copy Prince lyrics over and over again, inscribing coffee and starfish and butterscotch clouds. Me and my friends, in our flannel jackets and baseball hats and ripped jeans, dipping Skoal, laughing till we almost fall out of the sky—we all want the same thing: to set our minds free, to be wild. To become shooting stars, to grow fangs and run through the night, to be loved, to be crazy. We're at that age when every molecule of us seems to be on fire. We make do with reading Charles Bukowski and Anaïs Nin and comic books, we make do with joking and teasing, with recording endless mix tapes of the Rolling Stones and Bad Brains and Joan Jett, we make do with being nerds, being awkward, but being true friends to one another. Nothing matters but the blue-sky afternoon.

When I turn twenty-three, I'm getting my master's degree in writing at the University of Michigan, obsessed with writing and with books and wanting to do nothing else with my life but write, and at night to make money I work at a jazz club called the Bird of Paradise. Late afternoon, at the start of my shift there, the vacuum leaves the worst kind of bad breath as I push it over the dirty carpet, and the club seems depressing and small. At night, when the musicians load in, the jazz fiends sit at the little round tables with the pink tablecloths, and the other waitress and I start delivering drinks, candles lit, the bass player now warming up—the place becomes euphorically magical. I actually am not a very good waitress, because I get lost, staring at the trio, who themselves are lost in the song, playing something from John Coltrane or Sarah Vaughan. *This,* I realize, this is where wildness lives. This is how one gets to lose one's mind, to be free, to be ferociously awake. In this dark, glittering room, with artists, with listeners, everyone hushed, sweating, smoking—being together in the moment.

Let's jump to another club—Bungalow 8, in New York City. Downtown, west side. I'm thirty and I just published my first novel, the one I wrote at night while I worked odd jobs in Manhattan. Tonight is my publication party, and people are here at this bar to dance, drink, flirt, laugh, and help me celebrate. This is a dream come true, isn't it? Better than anything I could have ever imagined? And I do feel so lucky and grateful and happy, don't I? But I also feel like there's a glass wall between me and everyone else, like I'm a fish in a tank, or they're fish in a tank and I'm outside, because I can't *quite* make contact with anyone. I have an idea by now of what's gone wrong. My awareness of the problem has been creeping up when my guard is down: at some point in the past decade, I fused liquor and chemicals into my recipe for what makes me feel ecstatic. Various substances, too much and too often. And they do, they do heat up my blood, they make diamonds in my mind, they heighten life, for a minute. There's wildness—wait—now it's gone. And in the mornings, I'm deader than ever before. And alone.

And then, at thirty-eight, I move to Texas, hoping—in the back, silent part of my mind—to leave behind some of my habits. My house is an old bungalow, the yard rich with roses, jalapeño plants, amaryllis, banks of jasmine. The perfume of a new place. Standing in my garden, the golden morning touches my face like a mother's hand, telling me I could be happy here, I should feel welcome here. And I do sink into the city, and I do have fun, and I love this new world of cowboys and motorcycles and dance halls and unapologetically original people. But what else do I do? What I've always done, assuming it's the thing to do. And now, a few months in, here it is 8:00 a.m.—yet again—and I'm at the bar where I've been for fourteen hours, some part of my heart still somehow convinced that it can find wildness, aliveness, truth, realness at yet another dawn like this, with substances like this. I'm with a crew of folks who are magnificent souls—we're all friends, but really, truly, at that hour, everyone is a stranger; even I'm a stranger to myself. The morning light is raw and evil, the birds are cruel. I find my way to my bed, sleep the day away, again. And I wake up and point to myself in the mirror and say, *Please don't do that again.* And then I go out and I do it again.

'm forty-one, a volunteer being processed into a women's prison in Texas to attend the graduation ceremony for a writing program there. No phones allowed inside, no wallets, no pens, no lip balm— nothing but ourselves. They take our IDs at Central Control. The walls are painted with murals, and the place smells of cheap disinfectant, and beans and rice. We congregate in the gym, no AC, a fan turning slowly, and when I move my folding chair, the squeal of its leg against the floor echoes around the giant room. The incarcerated women file in, wearing uniforms, and we look at them and they look at us. No bodily contact allowed.

It's been almost two years of sobriety for me, and I see everything from a different angle now, but I'm not sure how to see this day. Never been inside a prison. Don't know anyone here. The head facilitator for the program stands—microphone screeches—and she introduces the first speaker.

The woman gets up—white sneakers, a loose-leaf page carved with ballpoint ink trembling visibly in her hands—and clears her throat; we wait, a cough from the crowd, silence. And then the woman speaks, tells us—through dirt bikes and big brothers and ice cream and first love and three-legged cats and grandmothers and car accidents and fights and kitchen jobs and childbirth and Valentine's cards and loans—her story. And my heart is pounding, the room is humid with life, thick, hot; it's sweaty; it's muggy with the realization that we do know one another after all, every one of us knows the other.

Forty-six years old, with seven years sober, and where am I these days? In an upside-down wonderland of highways and fig trees and movie theaters and hummingbirds and surfboards known as Los Angeles.

I don't know what on earth I'm doing, but I'm doing it. Gertrude Stein said: "You look ridiculous if you dance. You look ridiculous if you don't dance. So you might as well dance." Moved here with my man, and we live in a lopsided steel-and-concrete house next to Elysian Park, a lemon tree growing by the front door. Writing for film and television, collaborating with directors and actors, spending feverish days and nights working on storylines and characters. This place is bubbling with new art and possibility, ancient stories and mythological creatures.

It's still possible to be mean to myself, vicious even, about years wasted, not having kids, times I let people down, but I've gotten better at seeing through all that and jumping back to the jewel of the moment.

Pitch meeting today in a glass-and-chrome conference room on the twenty-fourth floor, and my nerves are raw. I'm suddenly telling this room about a dreamy, strange, dark story. It's like sharing a secret. Other people share their own ideas, coughing up stuff they've engineered in private and putting it on the table for all to see. Then the conversation rises and splinters and reconnects as everyone takes the project into their hands to weigh it like a new baby, name it, talk about how they'd raise it, if they were to raise it.

While the discussion evolves, I can't help gazing over the panoramic landscape, a zillion pale buildings, the palm trees, mountains in the distance, clouds that don't move. It's frightening to be up here, suspended in an unknown place. *This* is exactly when I feel that electricity, the wildness, the freedom. This is when I remember in the cells of my body what it was to be a girl on the foaming falling sparkling crest of a wave, to be part of the ocean—not at all fearless, not sure of anything, just rapturously alive.

DIVINE TRANSGRESSIONS

𑄳𑄳𑄳

I swim in a shaft of light, upside down,
and I can see myself clearly,
through and through, from every angle.
Perhaps I stand on the brink of a great discovery . . .

~JAMAICA KINCAID

POLAR-BEAR SWAN DIVE

n the past, New Year's Day for us was often obscured by the long, tall shadow of New Year's Eve. We'd wake up at 4:00 p.m., scrape off makeup, and limp to late-brunch-early-dinner with friends who also still had confetti caught in their hair and tales to tell—or we'd get up at an indecently early hour because the kids didn't have school and they wanted storybooks and rides to friends' houses, and we did all that with red eyes and our minds twirling with what had happened the night before. There was a broke-down glory to all this. It's an American legacy, to be destroyed on the first day of the brand-new year.

And we believe, to some degree, in the destruction of one's self so that a new self can rise into the pale winter sky, like a phoenix. But damn. Ain't there another way? If we're sober, do we always have to be polite and rational? Or can we still tear things up and turn them upside down?

An answer: the polar-bear plunge on New Year's morning. You wake up lucid and bright-eyed, aware that this is fresh time, the first blank page on the calendar. Your bikini or swim trunks are hidden under plaid coats and oversized sweaters, and you make your way with your favorite lunatics—or in perfect solitude—to the pool or ocean or lake, armed with piles of towels and wool blankets. You look out at the icy water, you look at one another, or you look inside yourself, you have second thoughts, and then someone grabs your hand and you jump together—breathless—wild—electrocuted by the cold—laughing—trying to get up and out, shivering, shrieking, and you wrap yourselves in blankets and race to the truck.

When you get back home, you make a fire. Every cell of your body is radiant.

Part of previous new years was the swagger and bravado after a big night, and there's nothing wrong with that. The swan dive into icy waters is worth bragging about too. Start off January with a little bit of masochism and a lot of pride, and eat Chinese leftovers or pancakes for dinner, and realize that you're not broken after all but stronger than you ever were before, and tingling, and ready.

MOTORCYCLE GIRL GANG

A couple of years ago, Jardine's friend Emily posted a photo online of herself in a helmet and leather jacket, standing with a big old powerful beast of a motorcycle—she and the bike were sparkling on the side of a California highway in the golden sun, and Emily was smiling in a deviously beautiful way. She'd joined a women-only motorcycle club, becoming one of a group of riders who lived for the road (one weekend a month) and took trips and camped for a night or two.

Jardine grilled her on the specifics. *Is it terrifying? Who are the other women? How did she find them? Who taught her to ride?* Emily has to plan the rides around work and can only go on weekends when her ex takes their daughter, which leaves a slim window. But it's a window nonetheless, and it's worth it to her to strategize. She gets the payback of blue sky, new friends with fascinating stories, and a spike in adrenaline. She sees new country, she tears through the hours.

This is one of those instances where Jardine saw what a friend was up to and it swung a door wide open. Maybe she won't go shopping for a vintage Ducati tomorrow, but the seed is planted in the rich dirt of her imagination. So interesting to note how role models change over time, how new possibilities crystallize. Jardine pays attention these days to the acquaintances and neighbors and coworkers who sneak off and do crazy stuff, sniff out adventure, forge paths.

We used to worry: *What will we do if we don't drink anymore? We'll have no one to hang out with, we'll be bored and lonely, left out of the fun.* But when we took off our blinders, there were people everywhere, hidden in plain sight, showing us stunning ideas. We just had to want to see them.

EMBRACING RUIN

J ardine's dear friend Justine has taught her many things—but this wisdom rises above the rest: an evening dress is more glamorous when torn from jumping a fence or stained from eating midnight cherries; and a party surprised by a rainstorm can be steamier and more divine because everyone is crushed inside together and stirred up by the lightning and thunder.

In other words, imperfection is enchanting. Too much control and exactness can sterilize the love out of anything.

The Japanese concept of *wabi-sabi* is something that gains traction for us every year and has particular resonance in sobriety, as we accept (and even embrace) the spiritual cuts and bruises we might have gotten along the way. The concept is more complex than this, but at its core, *wabi-sabi* refers to a practice of seeing every object as beautiful not *despite* the fact that it is impermanent, but *because* of that. An illustration of that idea is *kintsugi*, the Japanese method of restoring a cracked vase, for example, with a seam of gold, so that the crack will always be visible and a reminder of transience. The break is not something to hide. It shows the passage of time, and it elevates the object.

There are people who get sober with the primary goal of looking better. We are not such people. We're gonna be happy if we look ragged and torn by the end of our time on earth and we'll even be okay with living shorter lives if these lives are deep, rich, honest, bejeweled, shocking in where they've taken us, exquisite in who they've let us love and who has loved us, imperfect, idiosyncratic, even messy, even lonely. We got sober to feel deeply, to take risks. We didn't get sober to live forever but rather to feel alive.

NIGHT SKY

After years of staying up till dawn partying like maniacs, watching the sun rise now without anxiety is amazing. Never thought it would happen. Like a lot of stuff in our beautiful minds, the equation of sunrise-equals-sadness seemed to have solidified and there was no fixing it.

Ugh. Even recalling these memories makes Jardine queasy sometimes—that sensation of finally leaving a bar or club, way past its closing hour, and entering a grimly lit dawn, and getting into a taxi, somewhat mortified to be seen by the driver, suddenly depressed on a spectacular level and dying to be home, forced to see everything around her because the godforsaken sun is up.

So funny how something so gorgeous, something that can evoke spiritual awe, became her enemy for a while. When she'd be partying into the wee hours and hear the first birds start singing, she'd actually hate the birds. Who hates birds?! She'd hate the sun. She'd hate the day. One morning, Jardine arrived home in downtown Manhattan and had to navigate through an army of cyclists gathering on her block for an early morning ride. She did so with her head down to hide the mascara smudged down her cheeks and her psycho-pinned pupils. She hated the cyclists. She hated their bicycles. She hated wherever they were going to ride—and, mainly, she hated the lonely dank bed she was about to fall into, her own ride being over.

She told herself that her kind of ride was a fair trade—night for day. Wild fun for ensuing depression. And some nights were worth it, no doubt. And there were nights that were not.

It took years to love the sunrise again, to see it as something besides punishment, or a symbol of guilt, or a vague threat.

Now it can be a hopeful moment. A bath of light. And silence.

We've also found it can be a work period before the e-mails flood the inbox, when kids have just left for school, the house is quiet, and thoughts and ideas have room to spill out and onto the page. We used to hear people brag about getting up before dawn to write and we'd grit our teeth and smile and think silently: *Really? How wonderful for you. I hope you die.* Now we see that the very idea that *we* could change our patterns and enlarge our work-life twentyfold was horrific because it meant that every day that we did NOT do that, we were forfeiting something we loved.

Jardine has a friend—a tough dude, massive arms, beard, leather vest—who, once a year, drives to the Texas desert and sleeps alone with no tent for three nights to reset his spirit. He comes back and talks tenderly about being awake and looking at the constellations and the night animals and noting the smell of the air, dozing off and then waking as the sun starts melting the darkness on the long violet-black horizon, and how he feels a part of things again.

Jardine was at a writers' and artists' residency on a Maine island one summer, and a painter there decided to stay up all night by himself, and to wander, sketching and taking photographs of the moonlit woods and ocean and then the sun coming up and capturing how it changed the mood and spirit of the place. He was a minor anarchist, simply by going against the rules of day and night. And he felt dopey and silly the next couple of days, a bit off, discombobulated, his door cracked open a sliver to mysteries and new ideas.

DOWNSIZING IS PUNK ROCK

Amanda heard an author she loves, George Saunders, say at a reading that he'd learned to let go of things not meant for him. A simple statement that felt all-powerful. She speaks these words to herself every day. *Let go of the things not meant for you.*

Chardonnay, it turns out, was not meant for her. But what else?

Marie Kondo implores readers to ask if every item they own "sparks joy" in their lives. If the answer is no, toss it.

It's just so much easier said than done. We ask ourselves if old grudges serve us. Old fears. Old habits. Dear heavens, no! But they seem stuck to us like leeches. We learned a method prevalent in recovery: we note our resentments in detail, figure out the parties and dynamics involved, and then ultimately work to see *our role* in the situation. For some reason, that last bit is the golden key, unlocking the chain. But sobriety didn't cure resentments and fears and habits for us. It simply gave us clearer vision so we could work on them.

Sometimes, this process of letting things go can break your heart.

Many of us are terrified that getting sober will mean leaving marriages, shedding lifelong friends. Some of us kept drinking for years because of these fears. We had to learn to be brave, to tune into our hearts, to be willing to do what needed to be done, and to understand what was meant for us. We do not want to sugarcoat it: burning down your life hurts.

It can be worth it, though, and so sweet on the other side.

And clearing space often means making room for a new life. Many years ago, Jardine stopped in to visit Lizzie, a friend who saved up money and moved into a Miami motel for half a year with nothing but a bikini, a couple paperbacks, a dress, and one lipstick—to clear her head. To rethink her path. Jardine gaped, awestruck at Lizzie's punk-rock move to a vacuous room in a candy-pastel beach city, with no belongings, no *things*, to hold her up. It was just her, alone in Florida, with the sun and the ocean.

Jardine's partner, Neil, has friends who live in Sprinter vans, rock climbers who park near the mountains and move at a moment's notice. She also knows a couple who left their apartment and jobs and took their kids on the road for a year in an RV. Another family did the same on a sailboat for two years. Then there's the burgeoning world of tiny houses, with low-carbon footprints and a minimalist ideology about daily life.

This kind of downsizing has a revolutionary backbone. Because it's more than stripping away objects and debris. It's giving the finger to bourgeois requirements like a home with a two-car garage and pool, a stable life as a proper citizen in the right kind of town. Dedication to a midsized company for life. And those things aren't bad in themselves, unless our commitment to them is due to fear and being bullied.

We hope to live until the day we die constantly learning what to let go of and how to do it, instead of accumulating things and status. An honorable life in our minds would be fluid and even empty by its end, leaving more room for love. It can feel unsettling to sit in an empty space, in a physical and mental and emotional void. But it's just like how boredom gives ideas the room to arrive. The beginning part takes courage, and we remind ourselves that all good experiments take time.

THE ADULT SNOW DAY

When Amanda was a kid, growing up on the East Coast, she'd wait by the wall phone (her beloved "Big Button" wall phone) for the "Snow Day" call. For her, this hallowed day off meant turning on the TV, staying in pajamas, and gorging on microwave popcorn. There was no guilt or sense that she should be doing something else, something better. Maybe later she'd bundle up and make a snowman, but for now: cartoons and salty snacks. It was a *snow day*!

Now that we're supposedly grown up, there are still days we just want to get back into bed. Days we want to pretend we're sick, just rest. Eat what we want with no thought, watch whatever we want on our screens, sleep.

Part of staying sober is hearing the voice inside that cries for a break sometimes—from work, from parenting, from being a citizen in the world—and figuring out how to answer it. We sure used to know how to give ourselves a break at the company party, chasing and finding oblivion via the open bar. From the beginning of Thanksgiving through New Year's Day was often a very thorough departure from sanity, and, in many ways, we still totally want that feeling—minus the hangover and inappropriate blackout texts to a coworker and the dented car. (We still use the holiday season to let our minds wander into *what if* mode and think about having just ONE drink, and sometimes the best solution for that kind of mood is as simple as going to bed.)

When we need oblivion, or a break from the mundane, we can also indulge in an adult snow day. It's one easy way to be happy—taking a day off for absolutely no reason—but it seems so hard and illicit.

Once in a while—or anyway, *once*—just do it. Shed the shame. Stay in your pajamas. Say goodbye to your family, or your roommates, or your startup company where you spend eighty hours a week, turn off your phone, and lock the bedroom door. Slip under the sheets, courting dreams. When you wake up, read trashy magazines and watch *House Hunters* and put on a pistachio-green face masque. Amanda once spent an entire day reading and slowly eating a bag of chocolate chips because there were no cookies in the cupboard. Regular life will be waiting when you eventually open the door. But for now, play hooky in a snow globe of your own, the hours sparkling as they fall gently, uncounted. You're allowed to disappear. Isn't having jurisdiction over your own time the point of being an adult, after all?

We're going to make that call, just like the elementary-school principal used to do. *Hello? Put down your car keys. Got any snacks in the cabinet? Box of pierogis in the freezer? Some back issues of* Vanity Fair, *and a backlog of* Black Mirror *episodes? Better put on some sweatpants and a hooded sweatshirt, and hunker down—it's a snow day.*

MAKE AN ALTAR,
OR A MEMENTO MORI

A surprise-attack way to feel alive is to meditate on death. To make a memento mori (an object or altar that represents mortality), we collect a few things—a crystal skull, a dead butterfly, a peony in a glass bottle—to set up in our bedroom. An altar is a concrete way to cut through daily chaos and remember, even if just subconsciously, that every moment counts.

There are altars or versions of altars in so many sacred places—in meditation rooms and mosques and Jewish temples, and in churches and pagan houses and Chinese Buddhist temples. It's been a human practice over many centuries, regardless of place or belief system, to manifest ideas and dreams and offerings through tangible objects.

As Jardine sits and writes, she is looking at her windowsill, a space that was never designated as an altar but that organically became one. Pressed against the window are two black-and-white portrait postcards, one of Maya Angelou and one of Cookie Mueller. There is also a jar of ylang-ylang cream given to her by a friend, a tiny seahorse, her Japanese glass pens, an air plant in a tarnished gold Las Vegas shot glass, a ceramic poodle from the 1950s, and a vase her partner made when he was a young glassblower. Unconsciously, she has collected reminders of impermanence to be arranged in her peripheral vision.

Memento moris do not just come in the form of altars. Jardine inherited a latticelike bracelet, for example, made from the hair of an ancestor—a Victorian instrument for grieving. A skull ring is a memento mori. Fantastic works of art—from eighteenth-century Flemish still lifes showing a dead rabbit and a bowl of fruit, to Van Gogh's skull smoking a cigarette, to Georgia O'Keeffe's cow skull with artificial roses—are memento mori. They all honor evanescence as a pillar to our lives.

Beyond sex, beyond drugs, death might be the most forbidden topic in our society. Our culture keeps it wrapped up, sanitized, and far from everyday consciousness. This taboo doesn't allow the dead and the living to mingle, and yet we *like* keeping in mind that life doesn't last forever. When things are overwhelming, this is a way to remember that nothing matters except the basic stuff: food, water, shelter, and lots of love. A sense of mortality makes us reach deeper into the hour because there's nothing but the moment. How many times have we heard that and forgotten it? How is it possible to say it out loud but not feel it? Because it's difficult to stay there, and a memento mori can help.

We can use our homemade altars to meditate on anything we care about, not just human temporality. Sometimes objects and photos and flowers and feathers communicate more than words, so instead of writing in a notebook or reading, we can sit at our altar and be informed and get anchored. They provide sanctuary, a place to get calm, a place to feel protected. In getting sober, we didn't do away with a desperate need now and then for a place to hide.

MASQUERADE

As a tween, Jardine thought a masquerade ball must be the most romantic thing in the universe. Other girls were flocking to the mall and dreaming of more modern flirting and even hooking up, and Jardine (being shy and melodramatic and a bookworm) went for something more Venice, Italy, 1750. Before she ever kissed a boy, she had many a vision of castles, shadows, ball gowns, masked dancers.

A few years passed; she was fifteen when she finally "completed" her first beer instead of just sipping and ditching it. Beer was so sour and nasty, she didn't understand how people finished a six-pack. Then by eighteen, the reward of disinhibition finally became real, and she got over the bad taste. She embraced the magical properties of weed and booze, and magical it was: to put on a mask and walk into the night, present but hidden, finally able to be herself.

Jardine didn't get sober to spend the rest of her life transparent and exposed—that was never the goal. Especially for an introvert, going out into the world raw and unprotected is *not* the best idea. We all choose personae every day and night to interface with others, which isn't dishonest as much as it's creative. So it's not the masquerade we abandoned but how we used to pull it off, since that old method hurt more than it helped. Now we can do it another way.

Bring on the wigs and capes and wings and crowns, the drag and masquerade balls, the costume parties. Mardi Gras in New Orleans, Burning Man in Nevada, Gay Pride parades all over the world, the Carnival of Venice in Italy, the Mermaid Parade in Coney Island, Rio Carnival in Brazil, and any club or crew holding a dress-up night in your hood, or a cosplay birthday. Some people go to drink and get high, but costume parties offer something besides that because they're artistic and interactive, and you can hide in plain sight. (And some literally offer sober spaces—even Burning Man has recovery meetings throughout the festival.)

To reinvent ourselves is a primal urge. Growing up, we drew a mustache on our face with Magic Marker. We put gold stickers on our arms, and they'd fall off while we raced around the yard. We had a trunk of our parents' castoffs, their nightgowns and uniforms and straw hats and white gloves. We'd tie ribbons around the dog's collar and paint the dolls. Amanda's daughter spends hours in her grandmother's Savannah closet, emerging in legendary costumes and walking down her own imaginary catwalk.

A level of masquerading is accessible on any given day, taking cues from Rihanna's henna-Maori-hand-tattoo or Nicki Minaj's rainbow hair or the late Jeanne-Claude's flame-red head. David Bowie led the way with Aladdin Sane and Ziggy Stardust and Goblin King. We love the curated persona of Anna Piaggi, the Italian editor, with scarlet dots on cheeks and a blue birdcage for a purse. We can channel the genius of Leigh Bowery, or the master of identity-manipulation, RuPaul, who single-handedly brought the artistry of masquerade and drag onto the main stage.

We can just wink at posing or disguise. Streak your beard with gold. Paint fingernails black with glitter. Wear glow-in-the-dark sunglasses from the dollar store, or ask your kid for a temporary tattoo—maybe he sticks a unicorn on your inner wrist and you cherish it all day.

Masquerading triggers the interloper in all of us, that desire to hop the fence and swim in the neighbor's pool, to sneak backstage without a pass, to joyride around moonlit suburbs in our parents' car while they sleep. A friend found a vacation-rental fire sale for a castle in Scotland, and Jardine went in on it with twelve friends, and everyone wore tartan tights and black velvet jackets and sat around and ate wild trout and drank tea and felt a wee bit amused by life, and a wee bit invigorated by invading a different reality.

Amanda wouldn't even consider a Texas Book Festival Gala without a package of dresses from Rent the Runway. Once, her $3,000 Oscar de la Renta gown (Amanda's for three days!) was six inches too long and she ran to a secondhand store for mile-high stilettos—she toddled around, about to fall over all night. Then she got home, and the ball gown that had been amazing and impossibly possible and fairy-tale was suddenly a bummer. She kicked the heels across her bedroom and savored the moment of peeling off the dress, zippers and straps and ribs and pleats and all, since it was squeezing the very life out of her.

THE ART OF THE TOAST

Toasting can be a hard moment for a sober person. It can put some of us in jeopardy.

For example, we're at a wedding, and we let the server leave the flute of champagne in front of us—just for the ritual (we tell ourselves), we have no intention of drinking it—we plan to raise the glass with everyone else to the couple, but we won't have any. Then, cold glass in our hand, we *do* raise it, the world sips—suddenly muscle-memory takes over, and we're drinking.

Amanda has a sober friend whose *dying father* begged her to raise a drink with him. Before she knew what was happening, she was holding a cold beer. She decided *not* to sip but felt guilty even though she'd worked so hard for her 202 days of sobriety.

For people who are cool with booze, who never think about sobriety and don't need to, it's sometimes incomprehensible how one step can destroy a massive commitment, can topple an endeavor. But for many of us who have wrestled with the cunning and baffling force of alcohol, we know exactly what one sip can mean.

Toasting gives our sly minds a good avenue to get back to the old life. The social pressure to join this ritual feels like the law of the universe in that minute, and we must obey. But it's not the law of the universe, and we're exploiting the ritual to get out of the discomfort of sobriety.

Being okay with toasts has evolved for us into recognizing them as social practices that do have meaning, but the meaning doesn't reside in the alcohol. If we can locate the beating heart in a ceremony—which at a wedding is to wish love and joy to the couple with a raised glass—and we practice *that*, the nature of the liquid in the goblet doesn't matter. And anyone who truly can't handle us breaking from the small print of the tradition, even while we hold to the soul of it, can kiss our sweet ass.

At a dinner party in the Hamptons, Jardine was about to toast with everyone, and an older man in a cashmere sweater across the table looked down his nose and waved her away with his long tan manicured hand. *Not you, it's bad luck to toast with water.*

You know what else is bad luck, sir? she thought. *Being a dick.*

And thus she raised her glass to him.

PARTIES

Quite collected at cocktail parties,
meanwhile in my head
I'm undergoing open-heart surgery.

~ANNE SEXTON

THE VANISH

HAPPY BIRTHDAY, SOBER LUSH!

BRIDGE PARTY

FIREWORKS

RED BALL GOWNS + COWBOY HATS

MUSIC FESTIVALS + LATE-NIGHT SHOWS

COLD + RAINY MOVIE NIGHT

I DREAM OF JEANNIE

LETTER TO THE DRUNK GIRL AT THE SUMMER BBQ

THE VANISH

We thought of calling it the "French Exit," to lend it Parisian glamour. "The Adios" rolls off the tongue, or it could be "The Short Goodbye." An apt name is "The Self-Care Method of Going Home Early to Take a Bubble Bath Because You're Worth It." In the end, we chose "The Vanish," because, like any social butterfly with their own agenda, that's what we aim to do.

We had always surrounded ourselves with friends who liked to drink . . . who else would laugh and dance with us until the early hours? We tried to moderate *hard*, counted drinks, or only drank wine (or *only* drank vodka), or had a glass of water for every glass of wine. We blacked out anyway. We overdid it. We fucked up. The hopes of a manageable and harmless and go-home-before-sunrise party ended—more often than not—with a morning stomach full of sour displeasure, shaky hands, and a long journal rant about "not doing that again, seriously." Rigghhttttt.

Sober, we didn't suddenly let go of the party dreams; we still chased the dragon; we pined for that moment of glory when the whole room implodes into a sparkling cloud of connection and glee. (This was of course a rare phenomenon but had been the target for years.) We thought this joy could be found late at night, and only late at night: in the dim light of a concert hall at the end of a show, while sharing secrets as the bartender wiped the counters clean. It was the mirage of finding sisterhood at dawn, or rediscovering the early days of love while people straggled out of a closing bar. *Hang in there,* we always coached ourselves, *the prize is on its way, just don't go home, never go home, wait for it. . . .*

Then we jumped on the wagon.

As newly hatched soberlings, we feared being alone in the nest, and we feared the world outside the nest. We were still invited to parties and so we went. But we didn't want to be at parties sober and we didn't want to be at home sober. Everywhere seemed dull and colorless; we'd lost our known entry point to brightness and bonding.

Amanda remembers going to a friend's birthday party at a bar when she was only a few months sober. For an hour, she had fun, but then her feet hurt, and she couldn't silence the voice explaining she was tired. She missed the way booze muted these thoughts, and she wanted to feel simple and good, even giddy. But nope: she was worn out.

Contemplating explaining to everyone why she was leaving seemed daunting. She wanted her friends to know she was *still fun sober.* She didn't want them to think she thought the party was boring or that she didn't care about them. She settled her bill (one ginger beer, three club sodas) quietly, then hovered by the door. She remembered what her therapist once asked, "Why do you think you're so important that everything will fall apart if you do what you want? Let everyone take care of themselves and you take care of Amanda."

Would anyone know if she disappeared? She really did try to make herself stay. But her heart clamored to go home. Feeling guilty, Amanda jumped ship. She actually ran to the street, as if someone would stop her. It was raining and she stood under the bar's awning

and called an Uber. She took a deep breath. And then she vanished—
only to reappear in her pajamas, safe and warm where she belonged,
in bed.

The Vanish is a tool—a way to go to parties (or concerts, or dinner) but not be trapped. The only rule: *leave anytime you want.*

We don't have to say goodbye.

We don't have to be sick, have an early meeting, or feel a cold
coming on. What other people think about us going home is not our
problem, and a big realization we had is that most people don't even
notice we're gone.

It might feel very strange at first, but the *this is wrong* sensation
is a small price for doing what we want. We can bear this feeling.
When the night expires, when we're ready to be alone, we just hit the
pavement. We swoop out with the collar of our coat pulled up and
pretend to talk to someone dramatically on our phones, traipsing
through the streetlamp's light and into the darkness, channeling
movie stars of yesterday, and we smile once we reach the parking lot.

HAPPY BIRTHDAY, SOBER LUSH!

When Amanda had been sober for six months, Jardine stopped by with a box of handmade candy to celebrate. When a just-sober friend called Amanda to meet and talk about her desire to live another way, Amanda gave her bath bubbles and Junior Mints. Sobriety in the beginning can feel overwhelmingly like loss, so when we have friends trying out Sober Lush–hood for a pregnancy, a dry January, a week, or a lifetime, we love to spoil them a tiny bit.

A slice of red velvet cake or a tin of French hot cocoa is appreciated, especially during the first sober days. One fancy-ass chocolate in a metallic-lavender box with a bow can make someone's endeavor feel noted.

Some of us need to watch our sugar, so seaweed soap, wild-rose salts, and black-cherry lip balm are options. When Jardine told Amanda about a website where she could order itty-bitty vials of rare and exotic perfumes, Amanda found kits of note-centered scents to give to friends. Sober Lushes love a patchouli candle, or a Sri Lankan lemongrass or sweet orange diffuser. When Amanda prepared for her first sober Christmas, she opened a package from her sister, Sarah, to find an array of teas from Boulder, Colorado: white peach, four seasons jasmine oolong, Andalusia lemon rooibos. It meant a lot that her sister had thought about what a sober holiday would mean and had sent this in support. Just giving a newly sober friend a teacup engraved with yellow roses from the junk shop is a dear gesture.

We love giving short books for reading in the bath and on the subway and while standing in line. Jardine adores *Siddhartha* and antique pocket guides to wildflowers, or vintage skateboard magazines or *Vogue*s from the 1980s. Amanda gives her favorite copy editor's guide to navigating the beauty of language, *Dreyer's English*.

When Jardine sent her a gift card for a juice shop, Amanda made it a new tradition to share a mango clementine juice with her son before dropping him at school. These parcels are more talisman than merchandise, so a handpicked apple will do, as will a used Dusty Springfield album, a Jackie Robinson postcard with congrats scrawled to commemorate time achieved. And we believe in giving *yourself* presents too. At a Tennessee writers' retreat, Amanda's room had a claw-foot tub *and* a metal tray for resting a book. It was so decadent that she bought a tray for her tub at home.

We don't give gifts to "keep a person straight" or pressure him to stay clean—everyone is on their own path. Passive aggression could slip into showing support, and while it's really nice to have company in sobriety, no one owes us that. This often comes up when a group decides to take a month off and only half of them make it to the end. Live and let live, and take care of our own agenda—we keep that in mind.

What we can say is that, on the anniversary of our first year into sobriety, a $1.99 Korean face masque left on our desk (from a coworker who knows how important the year has been) can bring us to happy tears.

BRIDGE PARTY

Amanda's grandparents knew how to par-*tay*.

Hosting a bridge (or dominoes or canasta or mah-jongg) party, in their honor and in their footsteps, might fall into the so-uncool-it's-cool camp. Picture *Mad Men*–era women in tailored sundresses and jewelry, cinch purses resting at their feet; men slouching in suits, eyebrows raised, hands holding winning cards or canapés.

You can rent card tables or just push kids' desks together. Unearth your grandmother's tablecloths and re-create centerpieces of irises or mauve roses. On chilly afternoons, Amanda's grandmother served pots of hot tea with sugar cubes and lemon, and on summer days, she made lemonade or homemade fruit punch with canned pineapple cubes floating at the top.

Focus on foods someone can eat with one hand—nobody wants to stop playing. Amanda loves Wonder-bread pimiento-cheese or egg salad or cucumber-and-cream-cheese sandwiches. As a nod to Nantucket friends, Triscuits and cheddar on a tray. Inspired by friends in the Deep South, fried okra, pickled shrimp, and little chicken-waffle sliders. Miniature anything, in fact: tiny cheeseburgers, pigs in blankets, cake pops. Crudité is keen, especially those supermarket black olives, with toasted pecans as a footnote.

Anything speared with a toothpick is more exciting than anything not speared with a toothpick.

So-called Bridge Mix is traditionally nuts mixed with chocolate, but Amanda also loves Chex Mix and salty peanuts. If you've got crystal dishes, now is the time to use them. If you don't, now is the time to hit the Goodwill.

Even losing hands can look forward to cookies, petit fours, and cupcakes. Amanda buys a big box of chocolates and arranges them on a platter. (She also heats up grocery store appetizers . . . her grandmother would not approve but might just understand!)

The best part of a bridge party is having a reason to connect, a commitment to leisurely hours. We see it everywhere: a nucleus of energy created by a few people sitting over a game. Whether it's speed chess in Central Park, dominoes in Havana, mah-jongg in San Francisco, or bingo in Texas, we like to watch people play.

In Italy, Jardine hiked into a little town by the sea, and there in the main square was a group of sun-weathered white-haired men around a table, smoking, playing cards. What game she couldn't tell, and she barely understands Italian so she didn't know what they were saying, but she knew without anyone having to tell her a thing that they were lifelong friends.

FIREWORKS

The Fourth of July always meant two things to Amanda: fireworks and beer. Whether she was setting off the "Kid Rambo" in New Orleans' Bywater neighborhood (and then running from the police), riding shotgun in a 1972 Landcruiser into the Colorado mountains, or lounging on a beach somewhere, the drinks started early and the fireworks were big.

At least, Amanda thought they were big. Weren't they big? To be honest, on July 5, she couldn't quite remember. The best part was always the lead-up—visiting the fireworks stores hopped up on anticipation, a pocket full of cash to burn—and the stories afterward. The actual events were often blurry.

And as she grew older and had children, her thrills seemed less fun and more . . . well . . . dumb. By the time she got sober, Amanda was ready for a change. On her first clean Fourth of July, Amanda stayed home rather than run with the pack. She invited some favorite cousins over and spread blankets on the lawn. After dinner, they bundled up against the Colorado chill, lay down, and watched the stars. Instead of drinking beer, they drank nothing. They talked.

Many holidays have to be rejiggered to work better, but sometimes, the exact same fireworks just seem brighter when your brain isn't numb. It's hard to overstate how impossible this had once seemed: spending a night lying on a blanket, sober, talking. It was only when the alternative became bad enough that Amanda decided to try it.

On that first sober Fourth of July, Amanda was laughing when, with a deafening crack, the town fireworks show exploded over her head. Amanda looked up, and it was as if she'd never seen them before: the colors were glorious, the patterns astonishing, the whole spectacle so incredible she almost started crying. She had dulled them all these years, she realized.

"Mommy!" cried Amanda's daughter, twirling on her lawn, "Look! It's the fireworks!"

"I'm here," said Amanda.

RED BALL GOWNS
+ COWBOY HATS

We've always been secondhand-store fans (since our very first ninth-grade Greenwich Village hunting-gathering expeditions for used military jackets and vintage concert T-shirts). We thought then that things were better if they didn't come straight from the factory, and we still do. Jardine's Gucci loafers from the resale shop in Charleston, South Carolina, are *more* fabulous for their unknown but imagined past owner's history of yacht races and golf lunches and dramatic divorces. Amanda occasionally spends evenings with her kids at a thrift store, always coming home with paperback books and once in a while hitting the jackpot (*hello, buttersoft Coach purse for two dollars!*).

Swap meets are the next level of such foraging, and they can be even more bonding because they involve *trading* goods.

Jardine has hosted and attended clothing swaps, and *loves* them. Someone invites people over and tells everyone to bring anything they want to purge from their closet, and a platter of cherries and goat cheese and crackers is served with a tray of cold lemonade-fizz, and the clothes are laid out all over the furniture. The guests circulate gold kimonos and overalls and white cowboy boots that are beautiful but pinch their current owner's pinkie toe. One dear friend brings her very tall daughter who fits into the castoffs of another very, very tall friend, and they're all happy. Ladies get undressed and get dressed, shy and playful, peeking in the mirror, turning this way then that way, and someone finally tries on the red ball gown that looks silly on every single person here and yet looks divine on her, like she was born to wear it (Cinderella-slipper style), and the whole party says: *You have to take it! Find somewhere to wear it!* And people leave at the end of the evening, old baggage tossed, new treasures hanging over their shoulders (and they didn't spend a dime), and the host donates the clothes no one took to a women's shelter in town. She looks at her empty apartment and has childhood flashbacks of playing dress-up with friends.

Thousands of factories generate thousands of objects and garments made from synthetic threads and plastic and rubber by the hour. We buy things that won't last and can hardly decompose, cramming our world with stuff. Bartering as a lifestyle is not terribly realistic (feeding our family is unlikely by trade alone), but to swap is a way to taste the ethos or renaissance of anti-corporation activities like foraging, farm-to-table eating, or tiny houses.

This mind-set isn't new; it just predates the world exploding into industrial and commercial excess. When we got sober, and accumulated an extra jingle in our pockets and time to spend, it was easy to slip into buying lust. Better to trade, and more connective too.

Amanda loves filling Hefty bags with her kids' hand-me-downs to leave on the neighbor's porch, and relishes meeting up with her favorite kindergarten teacher, Andrea, who passes along sequined T-shirts from Andrea's daughter, Kasey. Another mom leaves Amanda's daughter Ugg boots, flowing dresses, *suitcases*, and clothes from the coolest store in town where Amanda is too cheap to shop. The moms trade photos of their children wearing each other's castoffs.

Jardine once open-endedly offered her writing skills for trade on Craigslist as an experiment in bartering, and was contacted by a graphic design team. It didn't come to much, but she got to hear stories from the graphic design team, who didn't actually know a lot about graphic design but had met working at a horse track in Florida and led a life on the road and had been in love for many years.

She also worked on a Texas farm in trade for produce, plus some eggs and flowers, as part of a CSA (community-supported agriculture) program. That experience gave her a tip-of-the-iceberg insight into farm life, and the artichokes tasted better than any artichoke she'd ever had.

MUSIC FESTIVALS
+ LATE-NIGHT SHOWS

n Austin, Amanda rides her bike to Austin City Limits, wandering from show to show, from a Danish singer-songwriter to a fiddle maestro to Parquet Courts, Florence and the Machine, Childish Gambino. She can stay a moment or for the whole show; she's allowed to float, untethered.

And the moment she's finished, Amanda vanishes. She finds her bike and goes straight to Barton Springs, the swimming hole next to the festival. It's always empty on ACL nights and Amanda gets it all: the moon, the water, the sound of Paul McCartney—*the* Paul McCartney—singing "Blackbird," his voice carrying strong and true through the air. On the way home, biking through a dark night in a wet bathing suit, Amanda feels she's finally found it: the place where she belongs.

On the other hand, having had music fest experiences that were pretty much chemical from start to finish, Jardine wasn't sure she could ever do them again. *Dear SXSW: I don't know if we can hang out like we used to.*

Even at a big concert, Jardine will survey the crowd and pick out the most shredded, twisted person there. *Oh—wait—yeah, that guy, he's gonna throw up*. Just like any veteran of the service industry has trouble relaxing at a restaurant because they cannot help noticing the four-top next to them has no water, Jardine can't help wasting a whole concert focused on the cross-eyed girl in the front row who has quite obviously taken too much acid.

She used to love seeing bands in underground bars. Walking through a room dense with bodies, everyone crushed and crowding, the music deafening—she loved the breaking of boundaries, the collective heat of a bunch of freaks who adore the same band. But these days her heart and brain love it, and her body doesn't. She loves the *idea* of it.

Same with waiting on line to get into a show, which once felt good, smoking half a pack in the New York winter night, talking with friends who'd been drinking partners for a couple of hours already in advance of the show, everyone loose and goofy, the cold air meaning nothing, bare hands that don't care, feet in block heels turning to ice and no one notices.

Maybe that doesn't go so well anymore because she's not twenty-two, maybe it's because she's sober, maybe it's because she just doesn't stay up that late these days so going to a show at 1:00 a.m. is bananas, or maybe it's all of that—but Jardine must honestly confess here that some things haven't been reclaimable for her—not yet, at least. Some things don't feel the same, don't quite work like they used to, and she'd be lying if she pretended this didn't break her heart. That's life though, right? It's a give-and-take. It's sort of exciting to admit that, to let go of wanting everything or expecting everything. There's dignity in surrender sometimes.

As with everything else, this is not to say that late-night punk shows aren't for sober people. She's known Straight Edge friends who've never done it any other way, who are night owls, who live for the mosh pit and go to three midnight shows a week. We can all keep one another really good warm company in sobriety, but it's a private journey to discover exactly what each of us wants more of and less of as individuals. No way in but through.

COLD + RAINY MOVIE NIGHT

We used to hostess, swanning around our houses, making sure everyone was fine—even if *we* were not fine. In our new lives, at first, we tried to keep the same gatherings going, pouring Perrier into crystal champagne flutes and pretending we weren't sleepy by 10:00 p.m. But we were soon looking for new ways to party.

One idea came to Amanda when her daughter pointed to a movie that was finally going to be streaming: *Born in China*. "The panda bear movie!" she cried.

Energized, Amanda sent out invitations. She ordered Chinese food to be delivered. She bought gold chopsticks and bowls for soy sauce. Friends gathered and feasted. Some brought wine and beer, but as soon as Amanda started to feel nervous, it was time for panda bears.

Surrounded by friends and bowls of fortune cookies, she watched the movie. Her daughter sat in her lap, warm and transfixed. She wailed with delight whenever a panda tumbled across the screen.

Now we love hosting movie nights. We set out snacks to match the movie, such as spaghetti and meatballs for *The Lady and The Tramp* (or *The Godfather*), pastries and coffee for a brunch screening of *Breakfast at Tiffany's,* gazpacho for Almodovor's *Women on the Verge of a Nervous Breakdown*, homemade milkshakes and cheeseburgers for *Pulp Fiction,* or shrimp cocktail and Martinelli's sparkling cider for the Academy Awards. Of course, homemade truffled popcorn goes with any film ever made.

It turns out, we still love to party. While the movies run, our friends chat and laugh; they drink or don't drink. And when the credits roll, everyone gives one another a hug and a kiss on the cheek, and goes home.

I DREAM OF JEANNIE

A manda's favorite Halloween costume was Jeannie from *I Dream of Jeannie*. Her mother made a pillbox hat with a veil sprouting from the top, bought a pale blue leotard, and made harem pants and a little gold vest. Amanda wore sandals, and remembers dancing through the streets of her suburban New York neighborhood, a plastic pumpkin heavy with candy in her hand, feeling magic. The air in October was crisp, smelling of woodsmoke.

Many years later, Amanda had to note that trudging behind her kids, costumed only as "tired mom," gripping a to-go cup of room-temperature Chardonnay *wasn't* magic. Amanda was vexed—Halloween had moved from elated girlhood to wild parties in college and then to trudging and drinking. Somewhere, Amanda had taken a wrong turn.

On her first sober Halloween, Amanda brought nonalcoholic red wine to a party. All the other adults imbibed the real stuff, telling the costumed kids they'd go trick or treating *very soon*, then *in a few*, and again, *We'll go in ten minutes!* Everyone was in high spirits, snacking on appetizers and making giddy conversation. Only Amanda and the kids seemed desperate to escape. Amanda realized she'd always felt this way but had masked it with Merlot. She decided to make a change.

"I'll head out!" she cried, and she rounded up a crew of kids. Taking them by the hand (the older ones whooping behind), Amanda led the charge through the doorway and into the dazzling, buzzing Austin night. No, she didn't need a to-go cup. Amanda walked through the streets of her chosen hometown, the kids swarming like moths to each porch light and then back to Amanda, opening their palms and shouting about every Bit-O-Honey, tiny Snickers, full-size Hershey's bar! Amanda's daughter, dressed as Wonder Woman, was gobsmacked. "Every person gives me candy for no reason?" she asked.

"Yes," said Amanda.

"Yahoo!" cried Amanda's daughter. Her sons (one dressed as the baseball star Jose Altuve and the other as a hot dog) filled pillowcases with candy, which they'd sort and trade later with their friends.

For the rest of the night, Amanda felt eleven again—a genie who no longer needed her bottle.

LETTER TO THE DRUNK GIRL
AT THE SUMMER BBQ

Jardine had just moved to LA with her partner, Neil, and their place had a giant window looking over the city. At the house across the street, the guy had been prepping all week to throw a BBQ, and today was the day. From noon on, she saw his friends come and go, smelled food grilling; there was a bass beat. Seemed to be going great from her vantage point.

Then, before the sun was anywhere near setting, a young woman staggered out of his yard toward the street, tripped, and fell on the sidewalk. She was dressed up in dark jeans, a silk halter, wooden platform heels, but now she couldn't even get up off the ground. The man with her went back into the party and then returned with her handbag. He bent to her, maybe to ask what he could do. She had her head down; hand over face, she wouldn't or couldn't talk to him. An Uber arrived. The driver looked out the window, not sure he wanted to take her. The man on the sidewalk had a long talk with the driver. The woman eventually got into a kneeling position, and then finally was able to stand to be helped into the car.

Maybe we projected our own shame and bad feelings on the poor love, but this was an intense thing to see. Some people never get that f%+ked up. Or they had *one* night when they were seventeen, and that was it. But some of us did that way too often, or watched friends do it too often, and we know those feelings way too well.

It's not casual, to go through something like that, but our culture acts like it is. We're supposed to pop out of bed the next day and laugh, text about it, send a string of emojis with black hearts and clown faces. *Oh, I fell down at a party where I was meeting my date's friends for the first time. I was out of my mind, threw up in the garden. Totally humiliating. Hahah! Ain't life crazy!* We grow up thinking these are necessary rites of passage, to be performed many times. But somewhere along the way to getting sober, we personally decided it's *really* okay to stop being nonchalant about episodes like that.

So this one goes out to you, dear drunken girl at the summer BBQ, whose name we don't know. We hope you got home okay, slept it off. We hope you have an awesome roommate who cooks you an egg sandwich in the morning and gets you a Gatorade at the deli, and makes sure you know how great you are and promises you'll feel better tomorrow and finds you some good junk TV to watch and keeps you company for a bit. We think of you with a giant massive ton of kindness, dear drunken girl at the BBQ, even though you don't know we exist.

EATING

Pull up a chair. Take a taste. Come join us.
Life is so endlessly delicious.

~RUTH REICHL

HONEY

CHEF'S TASTING

BREAD

PICNICS, BIG + SMALL

SPAGHETTI + SHOOTING STARS

LADY GODIVA

THE ART OF THE SIMPLE PLATE

CHOCOLATE CHIP COOKIES

HONEY

Fireweed. Key-lime honey from Florida. Orange blossom. Texas clover.

It was a blast of pleasure to find out the difference between so-so generic honey . . . and the real shit, the gnarly and true stuff, the local non-homogenized honey. We thought, *What's the big deal, why does this jar of honey cost $8—so what if it's from wild blueberries in Maine? Is it really going to taste that different?*

Oh, my love, yes it is.

We don't mean to say that whatever you save by not drinking, go spend it all on these new fetishized food products. But a jar of dandelion honey from New Zealand will cost the same as a vodka-and-soda, and will last a longer and sweeter time.

There's a poem by Emily Dickinson with a line that goes like this: *To make a prairie it takes a clover and one bee / One clover and a bee / And revery.* The poet sees a trinity, this miracle of flower and insect and revery, and we want to see it too. Honey is the only food that never rots—how supernatural is that? If you add the word *raw* into the description of a honey, our ears perk up. And then if you add *whipped*—my darling, you're speaking our language. What is it about honey that makes it so transcendent? It's the taste of it, the nourishment, certainly, and the feel of it—the sticky slow dripping of it—but its allure goes beyond the culinary. In some ways, honey seems made from light itself, like a resin from the sun.

To take part in the process is another dimension to the phenomenon. One year, Amanda bought her husband a Groupon for a beekeeping class. After the class, Amanda's husband and son invested in full-body bee suits, head veils, a bee smoker, wooden frames, and 30,000 bees.

Despite a harrowing pickup, a hive was installed in Amanda's backyard. The bees are docile and fascinating. Two years later, there was a celebration after discovering the bees had filled a frame with honey.

But apparently, you can't gorge on the bee's first honey. That's the stuff they keep for survival. Amanda's husband and son installed a second box on top, and the theory is that the bees will fly up and fill extra frames, and these can be harvested.

Only when bees are sated and safe do they make honey to share with others.

CHEF'S TASTING

We feared when we quit drinking that we would have to quit lush restaurants with tasting menus too. And it's true that some tastings are curated around wine pairings, and so these are not necessarily at the *top* of our list. If someone invites us to one of those, we can decline of course, but if we go, we can ask a server to suggest zero-proof drink options, and a good server will. More and more restaurants offer tasting courses with nonalcoholic pairings, combining dishes with zero-proof house-made shrubs (gourmet drinking vinegars infused with herbs and spices) and creative, botanical, experimental elixirs.

But we've come to realize we actually adore tasting menus because of the way they can elevate a night, and bring people together as we try courses, and connect us to a chef and everyone in the kitchen, and add back the pomp and circumstance that once came from ordering bottles and coursing out drinks—the fun ritualistic stuff.

When Jardine got sober, she also fretted that not drinking would cut dinners in half: They would be less intense, less connected, and—literally—shorter. Because drinking gave diners an unspoken contract to linger on aperitifs, to space out wine during the meal, to dwell on after-dinner drinks with dessert.

Now, for birthdays and anniversaries, when she wants a "big experience" at a restaurant, she replaces steaks and champagne with some cult-following chef-coursed menu that will last for hours, that will feel decadent and celebratory. It's a great feeling to put the night into the hands of a chef's imagination.

For her mom's birthday, Jardine took her to a private *omakase* dinner in Austin; ten guests sat for three hours at a wooden bar, where the chef made each piece of sushi in front of them. He was funny and provocative, telling them how he developed his menu and where he traveled, how he grew up, what he learned in Japan, and details about how he was preparing each fish. Even though the talk was light, there was discipline and mission and intimacy behind the night, the sense that the meal came from more than just that day's fresh import from Tokyo. Everyone could feel ideas bred from generations of chefs, and from solitary experiments, and from books; they could see concepts in the wild thistle here and a grating of Meyer lemon rind there, in the order of pieces, in the gleam or matte finish of each ceramic dish. The guests who started out shy opened up by the time mochi ice cream arrived.

But this strategy doesn't have to be reserved for big life events. The standard prix fixe or early-bird special at many restaurants gives that vibe of connection. Jardine and her man go to a little joint around the corner that has a super-cheap and yummy three-course dinner every Tuesday, and it feels like Grandma's kitchen, the room packed with happy neighbors and good energy. They feel synched up—for a few hours, they're a little community in a big city.

This might seem like a bizarre correlation, but Jardine used to love the contract to hang out that came from buying a bottle at a nightclub, or a bag of drugs. It was a nod to friends—*we're in it to win tonight, I'm pledging the next six hours to you all.* They all felt it. What happens if your new nightclub is a teahouse? Do you get one cuppa with your mate, and then, fifteen minutes later, you're saying goodbye at the curb? Using chef's-menu nights to replicate that pact with friends is a weirdly good alternative.

But on another level, we don't need any props; we feel empowered now to loiter at a table, to say to a friend or date, "I'm in the mood for a long, luscious conversation, can we stretch this out? Can we order little plates, and make it last?" A zenith of sober life has been understanding we're not servants to some rule maker of restaurant life that states you are not allowed to linger if you do not have a brandy in hand.

Let's save room for dessert, even if it's just a bowl of wild berries with dandelion tea.

BREAD

The last scene from Jay McInerney's *Bright Lights, Big City* was instantly familiar when we read it—the guys still awake from a night of dereliction, the sun coming up, and the bakery simultaneously sending out plumes of fresh hot-bread steam, the smell of wholeness, goodness, promise. That scene was all about where the end meets the beginning. A ragged soul receives an elemental gift and is renewed.

Anytime we buy bread, we get a whiff of that bigger transaction: from handing over euros in Paris for the iconic baguette, to buying brilliant savory little ciabatta rolls at a tiny market in LA's Echo Park, to getting a plastic bag of homemade tortillas from a Mexican bakery in Austin. Even grabbing a Wonder bread loaf at a Brooklyn bodega feels different from buying anything else.

Patti Smith writes about having a daily slab of brown bread and butter with her coffee, at her favorite cafés, a habit as steady as the sun rising. Something about the brownness of the bread, the slab-ness, the thick slice of life—we can feel how it nourishes her, beyond her body, feeding her soul and fueling poems and ideas.

Barry Goldensohn, a poet and Jardine's professor at Skidmore, always served homemade soup and local bread at their weekly writing workshop, which took place in his kitchen. He gave the students words from June Jordan, from W. H. Auden, from Adrienne Rich. He gave them time, and notes on what to change, prompts on how to think about their writing and new things to read. He provided a safe space to cut their teeth. He showed them ways of following traditions, and ways of breaking rules. The soup and the bread got woven into the rest, and she looks back now and sees his generosity through the lens that developed over years—she had to grow up to understand that what he did for those classes is everything, everything a teacher can do. He nourished them. He fed them.

When Jardine was living in a house in her twenties, a friend brought someone from out of town to stay with them for a few days. They all woke up to an ambrosial smell. This young woman, who no one knew well yet, had picked blackberries outside in the summer dawn and made breakfast bread for everyone. The berries oozed indigo through the loaf, and each person ate a slice with butter. They went from not knowing this person to knowing her very well in a way, caring about her, and after these many years, remembering her and remembering that morning.

All of these examples are meant to show how bread is a force, a primary component, one of the key ingredients to universal culture. Jardine used to think that about wine too, since wine is ingrained in human history in a similar fashion, playing a part in religious texts, in mythology, in classic literature. Wine's credentials as this pillar to humankind's identity used to be a handy backstory to subconsciously lean on when she wanted to convince herself *not* to stop drinking (in the godforsaken never-ending conversation in her head before she finally quit). Needless to say, sobriety won over Dionysus. But instead of dwelling on the loss of wine, why not focus on another profound cornerstone of world history: *bread*?

Jardine can't bake to save her life, but she's discovered that she can make simple flatbread from a centuries-old recipe, stay near the oven so she can smell it (since that is half the pleasure), and then eat a piece while it's hot, smeared with honey or butter. A quick bread is easy too, and doesn't require the mathematical measuring that most bread needs, so is therefore eligible for Jardine's oven. (Jardine *adores* recipes that say "easy," "simple," "five ingredients," and she always passes off the end result as "rustic.")

Baking, whether it's naan or raspberry-pistachio quick bread, is a sensual and spiritual act—the first whiff of it, the evolution of its perfume in the air, the sense that the bread is ready, the anticipation, taking it out, the sharing of it or savoring it in solitude, the way it cools down and the next day can be toasted and spread with jam or honey, and how it is at some point gone, vanished, and can be made again, from scratch.

PICNICS, BIG + SMALL

A picnic can be many things. We take our work-break sandwiches to the park, or pack a banquet-on-the-road for friends or family. We love thermoses of iced coconut milk with ginger, Indian quilts, and friends lying around and napping and sky-gazing together. We comb yard sales for fake-gold picnic utensils and big old wicker baskets with leather straps, foldable rattan chairs and old unraveling Persian rugs and a portable espresso maker (it exists and it's cheap and easy!). We love the idea of opening up a minivan at the edge of a forest and unloading a dog, a cooler or two, and a wireless speaker to play proper picnic music like Leonard Cohen, the Isley Brothers, Cocteau Twins. Amanda puts the contents of the refrigerator on a platter, grabs lemonade, and brings it to the backyard—*Voilà!* "Leftover night" just got glamorous. (And no crumbs inside.)

We can light our mood on fire if we combine the right ingredients: a cloudy day in Brooklyn, a curry-chicken-salad sandwich from our favorite deli, the neighbor's cat coming with us to the rooftop, purring at our feet as we look out across this majestic, sooty, enigmatic wonderland while eating our lunch and sipping an ice-cold root beer; we crumple our sandwich paper and gaze at the cityscape some more. We go back down, and the day has a spark now, an ember. We didn't sleepwalk through the work hours. We kindled a little time for ourselves.

So many weekend evenings in our lives, when there was time to go out and do something, we stayed home. We didn't want to worry about driving; it was too hot to be outside; it was too cold to be outside. There were bugs, crowds, traffic. We believed our excuses, but we see in hindsight that often it was just plain old easier to stay home and drink.

Sure, we love our cozy nests, but a summer night (or even a brilliant, sunny winter day) calls for venturing forth. We scan community listings for free outdoor concerts and take note whenever we drive past a potential picnic spot, from a tiny public beach to a lakeside lawn to a park.

It's extravagant to pack food you wouldn't normally serve outside, like grilled shrimp (cooked the night before and served cold, with yogurt dip), sliced pork tenderloin, or pineapple spears. Smoked oysters in a tin can are skewered with a toothpick, and you feel like Ernest Hemingway. We like to bring ingredients to make sandwiches at the beach, bags of chips we ate when we were little, hot sauce, pickles. A portable backgammon board, a few magazines.

Amanda's mother-in-law, a Montana native, is the queen of mountain picnics. She brings forks, knives, and spoons rolled in cloth napkins. Whether it's tomato and basil from her garden served with fresh mozzarella, and sun tea with mint, or ripe peaches, somehow unbruised and unveiled just as the crew reaches Ice Lake in Colorado, she makes every outing grand. (And the peach containers, once emptied, can hold foraged mushrooms to be sautéed for dinner that night.) She has even been known to bring a candelabra.

Bagel sandwiches hold up well on long hikes, as do spiced peanuts, marinated cauliflower, and salami, ready to be sliced with your Swiss Army Knife as you meander among wildflowers.

SPAGHETTI + SHOOTING STARS

J ardine used to think the pinnacle of culinary experiences mandated wine and alcohol being part of the menu; this, she said to herself, wasn't navigable; this part of sobriety would be a sacrifice, plain and simple. All her meals now would be inferior to past meals with wine. Period.

She changed her mind as she had beautiful meals minus liquor and somehow didn't die of displeasure. She realized that many meals in the past, in fact, had been marred by her thinking too much about how little wine was left in the bottle and wondering if her hosts would open another (*they'd better!*), or thinking about how much she'd already drank and if she could drive home because she needed her car bright and early the next day, or focusing on how drunk the host was and how mean she was now being to her girlfriend and how uncomfortable things had become. This is not to say that wine makes a dinner miserable, just that it's not fair to say that wine makes a dinner perfect.

Jardine had a revelation about all this when she least expected it. One winter, she and Neil, his brother Chris, and Chris's husband,

John, went on a five-day camping trip in Big Bend, a national park in Texas so wild and empty, they felt like the only people on Earth. They did a massive hike one day, twelve hours round-trip, and it was really cold on the way down. They stumbled back to their site, starving, and quickly—with cold fingers—prepared that night's (very simple) repast. They lit the camping stoves and boiled the pasta and heated up the tomato sauce and opened the Parmesan. They guzzled air-temperature water and sat in the dark and devoured their meals with headlamps illuminating their bowls. There are no words for how delicious it was—it was delectable, scrumptious, succulent. The sky over Mexico and Texas was velvet-black, and she could see a shooting star every few minutes if she looked up. The air was crisp as a razor. She was with people she loved, and endorphins were flooding everyone's systems. Everything they did that day cost so little, but they put so much into it, and got out even more.

This dinner-in-the-desert came to mind at a book reading recently. The writer was told by his editor that the ending to the manuscript he'd been working on for years wasn't right, that it ruined the book. Devastated, he tried and tried to figure out a better ending. Then he had an epiphany when he suddenly saw that the ending was necessary and important, but the rest of the story wasn't living up to it. The narrative wasn't earning its conclusion. So he rewrote the whole book—except the ending, which finally made sense.

And then he won the Pulitzer Prize.

It's vital to listen to the generous wisdom of your peers, but we always have to—*get to*—write our own stories. Sometimes it makes sense to change the meal; sometimes we change the hunger itself.

LADY GODIVA

iquor is called "liquid courage" when it comes to sex and love, but there are lots of aphrodisiacs besides liquor. People have been eating or drinking things to jump-start the libido for thousands of years, in hundreds of ways, in every part of the world.

Certain ingredients literally heat us up. From wasabi to Serrano peppers to sriracha to raw garlic to piri piri to Chinese ginger to rose harissa to cayenne to Thai chilies to horseradish. These oils and powders get the blood flowing.

Others are, um, visually suggestive. Let's say, bananas. And figs, especially overripe ones that are bursting at the seams and leaking wet sugar. Okay, let's just add all fruit that is overripe, shall we? We've also got asparagus. Steamed clams. Artichokes for how they open to the heart. Cucumbers.

Herbs and spices, those evocative elements, torn and minced and ripped and savored! Anise, basil, bay leaf, capers, cardamom, cinnamon, curry powder, fenugreek, ginger, lavender, lemon balm, mint, mustard, nutmeg, oregano, saffron, sage, tarragon, thyme, turmeric, vanilla. We can't vouch for the libidinal science of any of these, but we've been transported by the fragrance of them all.

And there's Jardine's guilty nasty favorites, like whipped cream from the can, green-apple Blow Pops, maple syrup from the bottle from someone else's fridge when they aren't looking, raw steak, eggnog (more on that in the "In Your Glass" chapter, including a short meditation on how wonderfully disgusting eggnog is), and the fried grasshoppers she ate with her man at a Oaxacan restaurant in Los Angeles (during grasshopper season, of course). Neil also likes fermented food, and has kimchi for lunch every single day. Jardine—even though she doesn't join in—appreciates the appeal, the idea that the food is alive, is changing, and considers all fermented food aphrodisiacal.

Isabel Allende begins her great book *Aphrodite* on the subject: "I repent of my diets, the delicious dishes rejected out of vanity, as much as I lament the opportunities for making love that I let go by." The art of the aphrodisiac is letting go of composure, trying the unknown, indulging transparently.

And everyone's aphrodisiacs will be different. Allende loves hot soup, for example, which just puts Amanda in the mood for a nap. The subjectivity of aphrodisiacs echoes the best and also most annoying truth about sobriety: quitting booze doesn't mean we instantly realize what we love instead but rather clears the way to find out. And no one can tell us what we love. In sex and love, maybe it was easier to get tipsy and let everything happen to us. Now we have to take action, to figure out what we want.

As with all dream projects, creating an aphrodisiac feast on a Wednesday night can seem impossible, especially for those of us who are overscheduled by parenthood and/or work. Much as we'd love to slow down and spend hours listening to Coltrane and feeding grapes to our lover, we might just hold that notion of simple pleasure in our minds as a guiding star instead when we get into bed.

Aphrodisiacs sneak up on you too: one Sunday you might get

obscenely triggered by this omelet with fresh butter and salmon, rye bread, and a dish of cold sour cream, and you and your mate go upstairs after breakfast. Or you try lily bulbs at a Cantonese spot and get a gleam in your eye. It could be a superrich ramen broth or killer mole sauce, a black oily pile of caviar at someone's engagement party, a first-date-at-her-house where she makes you risotto with truffles—and you're off to the races. We can replace the buzz of alcohol and drugs with every lick of pleasure. And even though we can't quote a doctor on all this, we think everyone agrees on the crown jewel: the oyster.

Raw, of course.

THE ART OF THE SIMPLE PLATE

Jardine found herself, during a rush of work deadlines, living off CLIF Bars. She felt like an astronaut—she'd always drooled for that weird cube of dry ice cream they gave her class on field trips to the planetarium—and CLIF Bars reminded her of those pastel chalky treats. However, she does understand that we should not live this way unless we're floating through stars in a tiny machine. When we're rushed, lost in work, or on the road, it's just easy to grab the easiest, more digestible thing around. And yet living on freeze-dried food is sad sci-fi as you find yourself descending peg by peg down the ladder of diminishing self-esteem. "Nutrition bars" are great when pressed or floundering for time, but if there's even a four-minute window, the small gesture of assembling a meal matters. It doesn't even need to be a meal but can be what Jardine's friend Emilia makes all the time and flawlessly: the Cold Plate.

The art of the Cold Plate is rooted in a Newfoundland tradition of a cold holiday potluck, while also riffing on antipasti platters and echoing chilled hotel buffets all over the world. When practiced at home, the Cold Plate has a lot to do with what's already in the kitchen. A slice of cheddar, some smoked almonds, and a green apple. Or pita chips and ricotta and dried apricots. A slab of refrigerator chicken, a ripe peach, and blue cheese. To be eaten with your hands.

Another version of this is the Minimal Warm Plate, which could be a thick slice of toasted bread with wildflower honey, or pasta with fresh thyme and butter and sea salt, or store-bought tomato soup with basil cut from the windowsill. Any herb grown outside in a garden, in raised beds, or in a pot on a fire escape adds to the Cold/Warm Plate life. So does homegrown lettuce, radishes, or zucchini, or whatever you can coax up into the world. A handful of ripe cherry tomatoes can be split open, sea-salted, and drizzled with olive oil in three minutes, and can extravagantly improve your day.

Look, we get it. Some of us are overworked. Many are tired, all the time. Sometimes we forget to eat, or only manage to make the kids' box of macaroni and cheese. (With two carnivorous boys and a vegetarian daughter, Amanda and her husband are often left slumped at the table after the children have eaten, their plans for an "adult" meal scuttled by sheer exhaustion or the need to drive someone to soccer practice.) Cereal for dinner is sometimes a thing.

But even if you're eating a leftover pizza slice, just pouring a Coke into a glass of ice is kind of lovely. There's something about taking the time to prep—putting your strawberries in a tiny china bowl with flowers painted on it, or even lighting a candle and using cloth napkins as you scavenge your kids' leftovers—that raises the meal. Amanda's grandmother's crystal ice cream bowls have made many an exhausting evening seem elegant: eating from a Ben & Jerry's container is one thing, but Chunky Monkey in a crystal bowl—*oooh la la!*

Our French friend used to look at us, his eyes full of sadness, as we'd stuff our faces in the car at the drive-through while *he* brought his white bag of food back to the house, put it on a plate, sat down, and enjoyed his cheeseburger and fries, then had a cigarette on the porch. Somehow his lunch was better than ours—not due to manners—but because he had space to appreciate it. That's all!

We made room in our lives by cutting out booze and drugs and the subsequent hangovers. The question becomes, What do we use that new time for?

This: *Cherries. A hard-boiled egg with salt. Smoked trout. A pickle.*

CHOCOLATE CHIP COOKIES

ome love to cook, and Amanda does not. Though her mother e-mails recipes weekly (the subject lines read "SO EASY!" and "BEST PEANUT CHICKEN!") and her husband sure would enjoy an elaborate dinner, Amanda finally needed to forgive herself for hating cooking if she was going to stay sober. Because the anger and resentment that filled her as she used to chop vegetables was only and *barely* soothed by wine. By dinnertime, nobody could thank her enough for her efforts and she'd bark orders about setting the table, glaring at her family during the meal, a meal which also never turned out right. And watching her family glumly eating charred pancakes was no way to start a weekend morning.

Speaking of recipes, wishing you were someone different is a surefire one for disaster. Dearest readers: It's okay to hate cooking. It's okay to order in, to give the kids noodles and a bowl of baby carrots. Sober lushes try out meal kits; we make the kids cook; we tell them to buy lunch if packing little Bento boxes makes us want to gouge out our eyes that day. We order pizza and read a book while it's delivered. Even someone who loves to cook might not *want* to cook if she's spent all day dealing with a best friend's crisis or a lover's meltdown.

If something stresses us out and makes us yearn to drink in sobriety, we pay attention, and change it.

No, as they say, is a full sentence.

Amanda's not interested in martyrdom or super-parent-hood. She's never even thought of the phrase *well-rounded* as a compliment. Being sober is like letting the sand settle in a glass of water: See where it lies naturally. Don't force it into shapes it can't hold.

Soapbox proclamations aside, Amanda does make peace with being a mom who doesn't cook by making one thing well: chocolate chip cookies.

On her deathbed, she hopes her children and friends will not say, "Wow, she sure was resentful about having to put down her *New Yorker* to get our Totino's Party Pizza out of the oven," but will instead remember that she was happy, she was present, and that once in a while, and only when the mood struck her, Amanda made phenomenal cookies. Amanda's secret recipe can be found on the back of the Toll House bag.

Some tips: Use Mexican vanilla, which you can buy by the side of the road in Mexico or most border towns in Texas, or order online. Fancy vanilla will come in fancy packaging, but in Amanda's opinion, the absolute best vanilla is sold at a roadside stand in Jalisco, Mexico. (It comes in a repurposed water bottle for $4 a pint.) Add 2 to 3 extra tablespoons of brown sugar, which makes the cookies spread out. Pull the cookies out just a bit early, as soon as the edges brown but when the middle is still melty and soft. They are most delicious when made with the help of others and should be served hot.

COPING

I wanted to be my own heroine.

~JESMYN WARD

PIÑATA TIME!

Whether it's Seder, Christmas supper, Easter dinner, a Kwanzaa feast, or Thanksgiving, when we dream of a perfect holiday gathering, we see ourselves with family and friends around a long table heavy with flowers, silver, ironed linens, plates, candles. Flames snap and crackle in a fireplace (though we don't have one). Someone—*us?*—has made appetizers from scratch, having risen at dawn to roast a turkey, filling ceramic bowls with French green beans and roasted potatoes and ambrosia (a dish Amanda's Savannah grandmother used to make, which requires painstakingly separating fresh mandarin orange slices, then adding coconut).

In our dreams, our families are intact and loving. Any orphaned humans, dogs, and/or cats have come for the dinner. The sun burns on the horizon; it makes us glow. Later, there will be toasts, laughter, three kinds of homemade pie. We tuck in the children, rub their backs, and then we will be tucked in, and someone will rub *our* back. We will be thankful.

Dreams of perfection are a shortcut to disappointment.

Holiday dinners can be a lovely tradition to a point, but they can also feel like strictly enforced conventions, gatherings that we must attend or die, and we even forget what we're celebrating. It becomes all protocol and etiquette, no heart. We've learned, though, that the holiday can be rebuilt from the ground up. Unable to make it to family across the country one Thanksgiving, Jardine stayed where she was and hiked a north Pasadena mountain, a bucolic pocket of nature on the edge of Los Angeles less than an hour from her house. She and her friends carried a picnic with them and ate the feast at the summit. The day was chilly, mist rolling and swirling over the city skyline, and when they came down, they went to Koreatown for yet another rich, delicious meal, with a different flavor.

We have vegetarian friends who make an alternative Christmas dinner ripe with local produce, grains, and home-baked bread. We have friends who take advantage of the time off work to hit a dream destination, and spend holidays in Shanghai, eating crab dumplings and sipping a nonalcoholic sour plum drink called Suan Mei Zhi.

Many of us are looped into big family gatherings during the holidays where the rules have been handed down through decades, and to challenge the rules would be to rock the boat, and sometimes we're up for rocking the boat, and sometimes we're really not. We don't want the attention of leaving early, or not coming—we don't want drama. Sobriety can be about choosing battles, deciding when to leave early and ruffle feathers, and when to sit tight.

And when to skip it *entirely*. We've got plenty of friends who saved their sanity by taking a pass for a holiday when they didn't feel up to it, when it felt too tricky, the family drama swelling like a ripe fruit. Lots of folks claim holidays are the biggest threat to sobriety, the most intense danger zone, so it can be good to think *way* out of the box. Centers run marathon meetings for sober people during the holidays, and there's usually a crew of friends throwing an alternative dinner or celebration if you ask around. We've had friends who took the kids holiday-camping, out of cell-service range, and did their own pure and chosen thing. Friends who established their own tradition of a triple feature at the movies, then dinner in Chinatown.

It's often invaluable to talk to other sober people as the holiday approaches, and discuss plans and weigh options, or even to text sober friends from a quick break on the back porch. The sober person can feel alone at a big table of drinkers, but there're souls all over town drinking pomegranate soda while waiting for Aunt So-and-so to fall out of her chair as she always does. Sometimes we just get through things, and we are grateful for that too.

Let's talk about drinks—to serve and to bring. One holiday, when Amanda was pregnant and visiting friends in New Orleans, she drank six cans of orange soda. Now, she plans better, bringing or serving a bottle of rose-lemonade or Martinelli's sparkling apple cider. We can mix a botanical elixir, something autumnal that looks as lyrical as it tastes, and put the pitcher on the sideboard and serve ourselves as needed, sharing with anyone looking for a nonalcoholic option. We might drink Topo Chico or root beer from the glass bottle. (Dangling a glass bottle from her fingertips makes Amanda feel happily reckless.)

Nonalcoholic beers, wines, bitters, and now alcohol-free spirits can go both ways for sober lushes. For some, the taste of these nonalcoholic drinks ignites the addicted part of the brain, and we steer clear. Amanda's fine with nonalcoholic wine; after half a glass, she usually wants something else and dumps it, but it's nice to have a sip or two sometimes. But when Amanda tried a can of a Bob Marley iced-tea concoction, she felt woozy and immediately wanted three more cans. She knew that feeling, and never bought the drink again.

One holiday, when a friend in Colorado offered Amanda a marijuana mint that "would make you feel like you've had two glasses of Chardonnay," Amanda did pause. After all, who didn't want to feel this way? But in the end, Amanda decided she'd sure put a lot of work into feeling OK sober, into hearing her heart, and she wasn't going to mess around. She'd tasted her true life, and for Amanda, it was so serene, so beautiful, that she would choose it over and over, even if it was often hard as hell . . . even if this meant never feeling buzzed again.

We can also answer honestly when someone hosting us asks what they can get or make for us. We initially balk and think, *Oh, we don't want you to go out of your way, please don't worry about us, we'll make do, yada yada.* But people who love us often *do* want to take care of us. Why should that be shocking? It's been a good experience telling our friends what we'd genuinely like to drink. And it's sweet if the friend is shy and doesn't know how to ask but tries anyway; years ago, we didn't know how to help sober friends, and sometimes, feeling cowardly, we ignored them. Props to friends and family who inquire.

Two of Amanda's best friends own a vineyard and adore complicated, delicious wines. When Amanda came for dinner one holiday, newly sober, she was almost moved to tears by the fact that her friend Drew, as he poured wine for all his guests, always returned to fill Amanda's glass with cold sparkling water. As if she were as important as everyone else. Which, she was learning, she was.

We plan now for what will make us feel happy and safe. We front-load the night with people who understand the situation, with a structure to the night that feels comfortable. If the holiday has *always been* one way, we take time to consider another way. We can say no to hosting even if we've *always* hosted. We can skip a late-afternoon happy hour that will make us feel extra sober and awkward, and start the event at dinnertime. We can be seated between people who don't drink much. We can ignore soused relatives, walk away, knowing their story has nothing to do with us. We can bring our own car, and when we're ready, vanish.

We can buy a piñata shaped like a turkey and fill it with candy, knowing that the best way to escape a tipsy table is to stand and yell, "Piñata time!"

THE PORCELAIN TUB

Once, a hotel room meant an escape. On book tours, Amanda cleaned out the minibar. One snowy night in Portland, Maine, she drank martinis by a roaring fire in the hotel lounge. En route to foreign cities, there was always a sense of lonely camaraderie at the bar by Amanda's departure gate; there were $7 Chardonnays in-flight. There was a morning in a room when she desperately searched through her memories to discover what had happened after dinner and found nothing but blackness, a void.

On Amanda's first "dry" book tour, she packed silk pajamas, a Korean face mask recommended by her friend Tomàs, and scented salts. She took the money she would have spent on booze and bought a box of Junior Mints, thick magazines, and another box of Junior Mints. It's true that she gazed at the people drinking at Chili's, remembering the ease that came with a preboarding beer. But she did not go in.

Another hotel was situated inside a shopping mall in Houston, Texas. Her room was large and blindingly bright but lacked a bathtub, and taking a long, hot bath had been something she'd been secretly dreaming about. She stared into the shower, feeling robbed. Her publisher would pay for whatever she wanted from the minibar, but what she wanted couldn't be found in a minibar, not anymore.

She didn't know, really, what she *did* want or where it could be found. She considered the gleaming skyline. She opened and closed a hardcover book of short stories. She was alone, but it no longer felt like freedom. It felt lonely.

She called Jardine and complained about the shower. She knew if she had to complain, it was better to share—it was wise and important to escape the familiar echo chamber of her discontent. Jardine suggested she call the front desk and ask for a room with a bathtub. She was not the sort of person who called the front desk. What she knew how to do was fix feeling wronged—all by herself. She knew how to open the minibar.

The strangest part of the story is how heavy the phone receiver felt in her hand. She held it for a moment, put it back down, lifted it again, and dialed. The man at the front desk seemed annoyed. Who was she to ask for favors? She apologized, stammered that she had hoped for a bathtub. Asking for what she wanted tasted bitter at first.

The man told her to wait. She sat on the bed—it was perfectly, tightly, made. She felt guilty. The carpet was lush on her bare feet.

A knock at the door. A young bellboy with a new key card. He asked if she needed help with her bags and she said, "Oh, no," though she could use help. She felt she had asked for too much already.

Her new room was on the very top floor. She rode up with her heart in her throat. The room was located at the end of a long hallway. She slipped the card in and heard a click. She stepped inside.

She'd been moved to the penthouse suite. It had two bedrooms and a living room with views of the city from every window. In the bathroom was an enormous porcelain tub. It felt like an answer to a question she was just learning how to put into words.

HEY THERE, BARTENDER

t's our high school reunion, our friend's birthday, it's a work group heading out after a long week, it's a wedding, it's a film festival premiere party, it's a fundraiser. And we find ourselves at a bar.

We've all been there, wandering with a crew from the twilit parking lot into a darkened bar, the group moving to the stools. Wallets out, that sort of dreamy and acquisitive look in everyone's eyes as we consider the options, scan the draft handles, ask for a wine menu. There's always the impatient friend who knows exactly what they want and they want it now and they stare down the bartender, money in hand.

And then it's our turn. After everyone has named French wines and double scotches and fancy cocktails, there we are saying, *I'd just love a club soda with a lime, please?* The bartender suddenly sees zero profit, and our friends turn and gape like we've just somehow announced that (a) we won't be having any fun tonight; and (b) we judge them all for their choices in life.

In the beginning of sobriety, Jardine cultivated rage: she'd place her nonalcoholic order, smile at everyone, and in her head, she'd think, *Don't f#$king tell me what the f@*k to drink or do with my f%+king life, you pieces of s*%t.* And honestly—that worked beautifully for a while. But rage doesn't sustain us, and isn't good for the central nervous system, and the bottom line was that she didn't actually hate *any* of these people, and didn't want to be angry each time she ordered a drink.

Amanda made her best friend order for her. She was too ashamed (in retrospect her heart breaks for her fledgling self) to ask for Perrier in a wineglass with a lime. She overshared, telling uninterested barkeeps about her last booze blackout. For a while, she stayed home.

We've already said this, but it sure does bear repeating: Simply not going *is* an actual strategy. Always. It's good to remember that even if it's our best friend in the world's wedding, if the reception will put us at risk of drinking, we can go home after the ceremony. Even halfway across the parking lot toward the bar, we can reconsider and say good night. (Or not say good night . . . we can vanish. We can. We can e-mail a vague apology in the morning. We've done it. We've called each other halfway home and cried and known we'd done the right thing, the only thing. We'd vanished so we could stay sober for one more day.)

We've realized, with time, that handling ourselves in a bar situation is less about avoiding alcohol and more of a case study in people-pleasing. There's still a whiff of shame around being sober in many circles, the raised eyebrow, the *why don't you just drink less?* It took us a while to accept that *it's OK if people don't get it.*

We've realized something about ourselves too: we are just as tempted by the propensity to make everyone feel happy as we are by booze. We want everyone to know we're grateful to be there, and we had to confront the notion that by not drinking, we'd be disappointing that friend who wanted a wingwoman for a bender tonight because she wants to forget her shitty week and doesn't want to do it alone, or that friend who's slightly sensitive about how much *he* drinks and is threatened by any notion that there's another lifestyle and that he has a choice, or that friend who (much like we did back in the day) had braided the idea of friendship and real connection into drinking and drugs, and so one without the other felt shallow and unsatisfying, like a half night, a dud.

We can't recommend one reliable way to go about the sober night at the bar, because it's so different for everyone. Amanda now opts for meeting friends for coffee or lunch whenever possible, since being in bars makes her squirrely. If she needs to be in one, she'll choose a bar (if possible) with charcuterie or decadent desserts.

But in case of emergency, here are some ways of being unapologetically evasive: you can always say you're on a cleanse, or off booze for Lent, or for the month of February (or April or November or whatever), or you're on antibiotics, or you're pregnant, or you're trying to get pregnant, or you've got a 5:00 a.m. conference call, or have some unnamed mysterious blood test tomorrow.

Some people drink nonalcoholic beer while others find it triggering and stay away, which we note elsewhere in the book, but it's worth saying again. Some sip tonic with lemon so it looks like vodka—a camouflage drink—and all the drinkers relax. These days, at many bars and restaurants, it's becoming easier and more elegant to order a spirit-free drink, partly because it seems more socially acceptable to have zero-proof options on a menu, and also because the mixology craze of fresh, ripe ingredients and innovative recipes from the last fifteen years has fueled possibilities in general.

In our current hometowns of Austin and Los Angeles, places offer drinks with fresh-pressed ginger or kiwi slices or hibiscus syrup, drinks without booze crafted like they're worth crafting. The concept of hospitality that includes sobriety has even spawned a new category of bars that don't serve booze but are headquarters for music, flirting, playing, dancing, and some established nightclubs and bars also do weekly or monthly nonalcohol nights. These are classy events because it's not just sober people who attend, and it's progressive and exciting to see sobriety invited into nightlife, and embraced by people who might drink otherwise but think turning their attention elsewhere once in a while is fun and sexy. What?

But at many dive bars, or even in an *oh-so-chic* restaurant in Austin where Amanda was informed that the only nonalcoholic options to go with her forty-dollar entrée were tap water and coffee or at the restaurant where she asked nervously for a "nonalcoholic cocktail" and was told scornfully that "all the *flavor* comes from the alcohol," there aren't many options. There's sometimes just gnarly flat 7-Up from the gun whose soda-machine lines haven't been cleaned in a decade and you can taste the gunk. As with everything on this journey, some obstacles are real, and to downplay them is not honest.

We can say this: over the years, *we've* found it gets easier and easier to talk to a bartender, to communicate what we want, to be comfortable saying it in front of drinkers, to pick places that work, to stay away from places that don't, to take a moment in the bathroom to untangle our many emotions about the whole thing (or at least to let them wash over us, storm on past), and to bounce back from the inevitable lame experiences where a friend says something stupid or a bartender smirks.

One night, at a fabulous hotel bar during the San Antonio Book Festival, Amanda and Jardine ordered a bottle of Perrier from a passing waiter. When he returned carrying a three-hundred-dollar bottle of Perrier-Jouët champagne, Jardine and Amanda laughed and sent it back but kept the champagne flutes, and toasted each other with water.

But it was hard as hell for a long time. We were beginners at something, and ain't no way out but through. The joy has been in building a new way of doing things from scratch, knowing that even though some people around us don't get it and don't want to get it, there are also many people around us (who we've found, and connected with) who do.

THE ARSENIC HOUR

Amanda's Savannah relatives call it the arsenic hour—anyone with small children understands this one. It's the hour when the screaming gets loud, when everyone seems to need you most, when a toddler smears jam on your favorite pants. Amanda feels that even when it all reaches this fever pitch she's supposed to be calm and collected—to cook gourmet meals and maybe even be a witty wife.

The sun is setting. She stands at the stove, wondering how she's traveled from graduate school to this kitchen, knowing she's supposed to "cherish the moment" and help with algebra and give her girl a bubble bath and feed the puppy.

Once, Amanda poured wine to stay in the kitchen. Life with or without children can feel like a slog, and sipping champagne while you do laundry can make the whole endeavor more festive. But we've learned that we can bear the tedium booze free. We can bear it, and it passes, one day at a time.

We can also, sometimes, say no.

We can open the door and go outside, to a hammock, or the front stoop. The first time Amanda left the kitchen during the arsenic hour, she felt both guilty and fabulous.

The guilt faded.

She closed her eyes. She listened to the cicadas or the traffic, breathed in and out a few times. Her heartbeat slowed. She stayed as long as she could, and then made herself stay ten minutes longer. An evening of cartoons and Fruity Pebbles wasn't fabulous parenting, but neither was a perfect dinner served by a woman filled with anger and Chardonnay.

We believe it's OK for the people who love you to know that sometimes you get tired. We think it's a great example to show kids that they can grow up to be people who take care of themselves.

The breeze was soft on Amanda's face. Inside, Amanda's daughter watched Amanda watch the sky. She waved, and Amanda waved back. The arsenic hour was almost over, and soon it would be bedtime.

This is what it felt like to choose herself.

A HEAVEN OF CHANDELIERS

On a whim, Jardine spent $25 on eBay for a tacky fantastical Dr. Seuss–like botanical lamp from the 1950s. Its base is a stem that branches out into green-painted metal leaves and white-painted metal flowers, topped with a moth-eaten rust-spotted silk lampshade. Turned off, it looks like a grimy object no one bought by the end of a garage sale. When she switches it on, it lights up some childlike part of her brain where fairy tales and comic books are stored. It also transforms the room.

SAD, or seasonal affective disorder—it sounds like a problem from an Ursula K. Le Guin novel set on another planet. Jardine spent a weekend in Stockholm in early spring, on a day when sun bathed the land again after a long, dark winter, and people went berserk—bodies out from hibernation, souls emerging from lethargy. We've had brushes with SAD, that odd malaise that arises in long snowy gray clammy months, but we've found it can happen anytime—as a rough mood on a dank summer afternoon or a struggle through weeks of rain in the Pacific Northwest or Cape Cod.

Light can take care of us. Jardine recently invested in a brilliant invention: the "sunrise clock" lights up a half hour before the alarm, washing the bedroom in a deep cherry glow and simmering into tangerine gold, then into pale yellow, and white, and then breaking into birdsong to effectively wake up her brain, which has been creeping toward consciousness, cued by the "sunrise." Vitamin D will also do a sun-starved spirit good. A friend who worked for Amazon in Seattle told us that employees were given "light machines" for their desks, which transformed the office. We imagined everyone smiling at one another, laughing, even kissing by the Xerox machine. And we have a friend who stocks dozens of black candles, burns them in a candelabra—it's a signature element to her home, inverting an early malevolent dusk into radiance.

Walking the grim damp New York City winter streets years ago, Jardine would sometimes pop into a lamps-and-lighting store down by Chinatown for a quick fix. The whole place was glittering, its ceiling hung with dozens of chandeliers—some crude like 1980s mobster-mansion lights, others fragile and art deco or faux-Versailles, some dripping with lavender crystals or red glass flowers. The place rained light on her, the kind of drizzle so gentle no one opens an umbrella, the kind that feels good. A replenishment to some reservoir in the soul.

THE BURN NOTEBOOK

When we stop drinking away emotions, some of us realize we're angry. And sobriety doesn't "cure" that. A Honda Odyssey cut off Amanda as she drove her children to school, and she felt a scream welling up in her throat. While doing dishes without the buffer of a few glasses of wine, Amanda felt an uncomfortable, hot fury. And she felt anger toward her newly sober, fragile self.

Sober friends told Amanda this was normal—they, too, had been surprised by their rage. She was told to sit still and let the lava burn. If she could "feel" it instead of burying it, the anger would have a chance to fade. But she didn't know how to "feel" it, and honestly, it scared her. For a few months, waves of anger and sadness hit Amanda and knocked her down, and not always at a convenient time.

She was angry that she couldn't drink. It wasn't fair, and many times she wanted to just pour a glass and to hell with this sobriety crap. She was angry at herself for the times she drank too much. One by one, she replayed these nights, her stomach aching as she berated herself—angry, so angry and disappointed in who she had let herself become.

She was angry about old hurts: childhood years she couldn't even remember, college mean girls, workplace slights from the 1990s. These old scrapes seemed so petty and useless, and Amanda was angry at herself for being angry about them. She was angry about new slights or imagined slights. (Damn you, Honda-Odyssey-man-in-sunglasses on Lamar and Barton Skyway!)

She was angry that there were no more Pringles in the Pringles can. *WHO ATE THE LAST OF THE PRINGLES AND PUT AWAY THE EMPTY CAN? WHO?*

When a famous writer treated Amanda meanly during an event, Amanda was engulfed by rage. (She's still mad, honestly. Why be mean, famous writer? *WHY?*)

A die-hard bookworm, Amanda researched ways to handle anger. Besides Pringles pig-outs and extralarge boxes of Junior Mints, she found some good ideas and tried them. She began with the "burn notebook." Amanda wrote down every rude, awful, frightening, angry thought that came into her mind. (Imagining the objects of her anger—even addressing letters to them—helped get her going.) She didn't censor herself. One website suggested using her left hand to access childhood thoughts. After she completed her letter, she lit a fire in her outdoor firepit, tossed in her letter, and watched it burn to ashes.

Next, she tried "towel twisting," grabbing one end of a big, fluffy towel in each hand. She pictured who and what she was mad at and started twisting. She yelled the name of the famous, rude author as she twisted with all her strength until her anger was wrung out of her and she collapsed, shocked and a bit impressed by the might of her fury.

Amanda also went for "car screaming," pulling over in a vacant lot, gripping her steering wheel, scrunching up her fists and face, and then opening up and screaming at the top of her lungs.

Then there's "pillow punching." Amanda knelt in the middle of her bed and started swinging. Yelling is a nice add-on to this method. As a bonus, her pillows looked pretty and fluffed up afterward.

Last but certainly not least, we hope to try "the big smash." This is an advanced method that requires preparation. At a weekend yard sale, we will load up on cheap glasses and dishware. We'll bring the stuff into our backyard after dark and take aim at our garden sheds. We imagine, and cannot wait to prove, that the sound of smashing plates and wineglasses feels even better than drinking a martini.

Once we learn to give the rage some room, we might see it more clearly, and we can start investigating its origin and its architecture. But we can't begin that process if we never let the anger out.

THANK YOU

Maybe we looked for reasons to drink. It's possible, and it works: a long commute, a loud neighbor, heartbreak, Tuesday. We decided we were "celebrating ourselves" with wine. Advertisements supported us, selling us "Mommy Juice Merlot" and T-shirts that read "I drink coffee because I need it and wine because I deserve it!"

Now, we look for reasons to be thankful. It took a while to shift our focus. Some days, all we can come up with is *I'm thankful I'm in bed.*

So we say *thank you* for our bed. A long commute allows us to be thankful for a podcast, for time alone. We're thankful someone left a book for us to read on our desk, that our brother called to check in, that the cactus flowers outside are blooming, that our partner cooked tamales tonight and they were delicious even though they fell apart, that our cat is curled up on our lap and purring so loud the sound vibrates through our body, that it's raining, that there's a full moon, that there's a quarter moon, that there's a blue moon, that we're alive. Searching for reasons to be grateful helped us to change the way we live, and the more we named these lovely things to be grateful for, the more these lovely things seemed to happen. A funny magic.

Some of us write "Gratitude Lists" in a leather-bound journal. Some have "Gratitude Groups" online. Some of us surreptitiously scribble gratitude lists on the back of a handout in a big blowhard work meeting that would otherwise catapult us into an evil mood. At the end of every day, even on the worst day, we seek reasons to be grateful. Mommy Juice used to mute our anger. Being grateful pulls our gaze toward the light.

LOS ANGELES WINDOW, OR HOW TO BREATHE

We have always been interested in the process and outcome of meditation. As David Lynch, a lifelong meditator, says, "Little fish swim on the surface, but the big ones swim down below. If you can expand the container you're fishing in—your consciousness—you can catch bigger fish." But we realize that to embark on meditation with a conquest in mind is to undermine it. So wait—how does this meditation thing work again?

Many of us are willing—or anyway, we *want* to be willing—to try but don't know where to start. We can't afford the time or expense of a retreat, and we're scared of walking into a class with strangers playing instruments and chanting, not knowing how to fit in.

When Amanda met Jardine, she had tried to meditate three times in her life: Once, in her car, when her daughter was late coming out of ballet class, Amanda closed her eyes and tried not to think. All the worries of her day came crashing into her mind with such force that Amanda opened her eyes and wildly looked around her car for something—anything—to distract her. Hurray! She found her son's *Captain Underpants* book and opened it, thrilled to have something to focus on, no matter how gross. And then Amanda's daughter showed up, with lots to say, and Amanda was restored to her usual state of feeling needed and overwhelmed.

Amanda's second attempt at meditation came during a massage her husband gave her for her birthday. Usually, during any mental downtime such as during a yoga class or a massage, Amanda assigns herself something to figure out about her novel. (Or she begins chatting with the masseuse, encouraging her hapless body worker to hand over all her problems so Amanda can happily—codependently—try to solve them in fifty minutes.) She now understands that this reflects her terror of her own resting mind, but it's also pretty efficient. Regardless, she decided on this one occasion to focus on her breathing and feeling the massage. This worked for about thirty seconds, and then Amanda began to worry about her children, climate change, and if something was very wrong with her left shoulder for the remaining forty-nine minutes and thirty seconds.

Last, Amanda signed up for a yoga nidra class at a studio near her home in Austin. So-called sleeping yoga, this class promised the benefit of eight hours of sleep in ninety minutes. Amanda arrived to a warm room overfilled with people many years her junior. Amanda (aping her classmates) gathered pillows and a dingy blanket and settled between a pregnant woman with awesome tattoos and a man with a man bun and beard but no shirt. Everyone arranged their pillows artfully, but Amanda couldn't get it right. Still, she lay down and listened to the teacher's soothing voice and reverberations from the gong.

Oh my God, it was hot in that room. Amanda began to feel claustrophobic, and instead of focusing on whatever peaceful thought the teacher was exploring, Amanda wondered whether the scratchy rug beneath her or the blanket over her shoulders might have bedbugs that Amanda would bring home, infesting her bed and her children's beds and requiring an extensive, possibly carcinogenic remediation.

Then Amanda began to feel like she had as a kid, scared and miserable, the words *I need to get out of here* clanging in her mind. She was near the window and, hot and panicked, she pulled the heavy (bug-laden?) curtain aside and focused on the neon gas-station sign across the street. She wished she were a stronger person and could get up and leave. But she was not, and so she lay there, sweating and miserable, until the class was over.

And then, at Jardine's house, Amanda sat on a wooden seat made by Jardine's partner just for meditating. Jardine opened a book, Pema Chödrön's *Comfortable with Uncertainty*, and they chose a one-page passage to read aloud as a starting point, then set a timer for ten minutes. It was wonderful to have something to orient her mind around. The passage likened emotions to clouds passing by a mountain, with Amanda as the mountain. It made sense. (So much more sense than "just think about nothing.") Amanda felt a rise of panic, a To Do list looming, but she knew she could handle everything in a few minutes. The panic lingered, quickening her heartbeat but then passed. After about seven minutes, Amanda was restless and began a grocery list. But still: seven minutes!

Friends have recommended phone apps that guide meditation— and give you the dopamine-producing thrill of an app besides. Amanda likes to pull a tarot card or read from Chödrön or a daily reader and then sit back for a few minutes and reflect.

Sometimes, she meditates to inhabit an experience. Sometimes, she's had a long day and needs to decompress. When she's stuck or panicked about work, Amanda poses a question and lets her resting mind answer. For weeks, Amanda forgets to meditate but then remembers. Meditation is like sobriety in that it doesn't make everything perfect but helps us be okay with how everything *is*.

Jardine was scouring the Los Angeles County Museum of Art calendar for free events. Mindful Mondays sounded interesting, so she went. A pair of meditation instructors took the twenty-or-so guests into an exhibition after the museum closed. Everyone chose a painting they wanted to meditate on and sat on folding chairs in front of their painting for twenty minutes, trying not to think as much as to focus on breathing and on what they were seeing. She felt like a *megadork* sitting there but then got into it.

Jardine thought she understood the basics of the painting within a few moments, her eyes roving, inventorying the canvas. But as she made herself continue to look as per the directions, patterns emerged, details and idiosyncrasies bloomed from the image. By the end of twenty minutes, she was floored by what she would have missed if she'd looked in a rush, or looked at the painting while also half-looking at her phone, or while stressing about work. She looked with her whole self, for once.

Then people got into discussion groups, and even the shyest among them had unexpected insights. Jardine's mind was turned inside out in a good way.

She recently found herself staring out her kitchen window at what is still a new and unknown city to her, with its hills and bougainvillea and chalky buildings. It was easy to slip into a place of loneliness and wanting, craving some sense of security or undeniable meaning, into that mood where she's sure she needs something and doesn't know what. And once she gets started down that track, oh boy, there's no turning back. Or is there? By focusing on her breath in that moment, she managed to let these abstract cravings fall away and suddenly—this is true, she swears!—she was ecstatic about what she already had and didn't need anything else. It was practicing meditation now and then over the years, building new neural pathways that allowed this reversal of a runaway train.

BUSINESS DRINKS IN MALIBU

D riving up the Pacific Coast Highway, lights on the water, mist on the ocean, her nervous hands are on the steering wheel. Jardine has a "drinks" meeting at a luxe restaurant and pulls into the valet, simultaneously excited to talk shop with potential collaborators on a TV-series project and dreading that moment, that yawning chasm of never-ending milliseconds of quiet, after she's asked about her drinking preferences— *Do you usually do red or are you a rosé type? Let's get champagne! This is worth celebrating. Who wants to join me with a scotch? They have a fantastic spirits list here, aged whiskey. . . .*

And then she says, *Oh, haha. I'm all about the club soda, actually. Yeah. So.*

And the table processes the news, their heads buzzing, faces unable to hide surprise (*huh, would have thought she was more easygoing, I took her for a person who really likes life*), and then they fake-smile, aligning against her, and the new work relationship goes sour, and her project turns to dust. . . .

This is the nightmare, not the reality. This is what she braces for—it's not what usually happens. But there is a kernel of truth in there, a trace of past experiences. Networking and coworker bonding and work retreats are so often alcohol-oriented that it's a big gnarly thorny prickly challenge for many of us.

One reason *we* find these work-environment moments hard to navigate is that our respective reasons for giving up drinking are hard to summarize. Each is unique and complex, would take hours to explain, and includes private material, so coming up with a sound bite to ease the social situation is hard. For instance—say we're at a Mexican restaurant and everyone is celebrating a big sale for the company and ordering margaritas and trying so hard to get us to join, and asking, *Why not just one just tonight? Come on.* What should we say?

I'm sober because a friend died of alcoholism and I decided to quit. Or *I drove one too many times in a blackout and decided to quit.* Or *My drinking was contributing to a slow-growing suicidal depression.* Or *I quit because I just didn't love it, and thought I'd cut out anything from my life that felt unnecessary. So no thanks. I won't have "just one" margarita with you, but I'm here, I'm celebrating, I'd be having fun if you'd stop asking me to break my private commitment to myself.*

And the needle goes sliding and scratching off the record. Silence.

Maybe we don't want any of those people to know any of those things, maybe we're not ready to talk about *why* to *anyone* at all, maybe we don't want to bring up serious stuff while everyone is having a blast, maybe we feel our reason for sobriety will sound like judgment of others and of their drinking when it's just what we wanted for ourselves. And yet they ask. They wait for an answer. Drinking booze is a social tradition, woven deeply into business relationships. They want to know why we just ordered a ginger ale. That shit is real.

We've often found the business-drinks-conundrum to be a game-time decision in terms of how we handle it, but it's a situation that can be very empowered by some prep work.

Part of the planning, of course, is micro-brainstorming the actual what-are-you-drinking element of the night. Options include the following: Getting there early so when they arrive, you already have a cocktail-looking thing in your hand. Murmuring vague statements like, *I'll start with a seltzer and lime and go from there*, as if you just arrived from the gym, and picture them forgetting all about what you're drinking as the night rolls on. We say things like, *I don't drink, but please drink for me, I'll drink vicariously through you. Or I don't drink anymore, but I still like to stay up late and go dancing, so don't leave me behind. Or I don't drink anymore and trust me, this is a good thing, but I love bars like this one and talking for hours, so my life is not that different.*

And then the other part of the premeditative process is parsing out what we want to achieve at this meeting. What we want them to know about us from the meeting, what we want to know about them, how we want to connect. This stuff doesn't really have anything to do with alcohol. Just like most business deals don't have much to do with the golf course where they got made. Golf is a vehicle. Booze can be a vehicle, but it helps *us* to think of a business meeting over "drinks" as the ritual of sitting and breaking good bread and talking and sipping something cold. The heart of the custom can remain, even if what we sip is a ginger beer instead of a martini. We imagine many a deal could be sealed on a squash court instead of on the tennis court, and it's the same deal.

But even though we've realized these profound truths about squash, ahem, the potential employer we're meeting might still think a martini means something that a grapefruit-and-tonic does not. First of all, if the boss and her workplace are supercentered around drinking, maybe it's not the employer for us. But if it's just an ordinary bias we encounter, we can start small and lie, evade, do whatever we want.

Amanda often feels most comfortable by texting or e-mailing beforehand, saying *Just a heads-up that I got sober a while back so I'll be drinking Topo Chico—can't wait to see you at 6!* Then she doesn't spend the evening wondering when and if the topic will come up.

All's fair in love and in war and in our first conversation with someone about sobriety. When we get to know them better and feel more comfortable, we can fill them in. This is the natural trajectory of any relationship anyway. We don't spill it all on day one. And then there's always the tactic of trying, at least *trying,* to shift the location to breakfast or lunch or coffee. We know, it's not always easy. (For sober folks who risk relapse in the presence of booze, it doesn't matter if it's easy or not, of course. To be safe is paramount, and so requests must be made to ensure that safety. We're speaking as two sober people who are able to be in the presence of drinkers, and our advice comes from that perspective.)

Jardine always keeps in mind that she herself (when she still drank) used to believe sober people were somber, overly responsible, judgmental, health-obsessed, that they didn't want to stay long at the table, that they knew things she didn't, that they were fragile, that they needed to be treated a special way. So she tries to go into business-drinks with empathy for the person who might say something annoying about sobriety or who just doesn't get it, since she *was* that person.

Jardine remembers one of the first sober people she ever hung out with. He owned a couple of clubs in New York City, and it took a while to even notice he wasn't drinking or doing drugs because he stayed up late, dressed like an outer space cowboy from 1978, laughed loud and often, and loved to dance. This was not the sober profile Jardine had somehow compiled from rather scant real-life data.

She finally asked him one night if he was in fact sober (and she's pretty sure she did it awkwardly and accusingly, as if inquiring whether he had syphilis). He answered with a big old grin: *Sure am. Sober as daylight.*

Why? she asked.

Because, he said, still grinning, twinkle in his eye. *I'm happier this way.*

She chewed on that for a minute, then he leaned over to conspiratorially whisper: *And it lets me run my business and have fun at the same time. 'Cause while you kids are spending all your money, I'm raking it in.*

He couldn't have picked a work-world more entwined with substances if he tried. He must have had to field questions from naive and clumsy and nosy people like Jardine all the time, and he did it with style, class, mischief, intrigue. He redefined for himself and those who got to know him what partying means, what having a good time means, what connecting means. He didn't act like he owed people extensive explanations about his choice, but he also didn't mind talking about it, and he didn't make inquirers feel stupid or ashamed for asking. She has a feeling it took him time, maybe years, to get to that point, to a place where he could be a king of his night and proud of his life without alienating people who live differently, and she hopes he's still perched on some barstool while a DJ explodes everyone's ears and lights pop against the walls and clumps of gorgeous inventive night-people orbit around him.

LISTEN UP

There's a voice inside each of us that we might call our true heart. Some call it our "inner child"; some refer to it as "intuition" or "a gut feeling." It's the voice that speaks when we are still, in meditation or in the moments after waking before we grab our phone to check the news or see if we have messages. It's the midnight voice—not the worry-loop one but the one that tells us we are safe and can rest.

Sometimes, the voice says things that are very hard to hear. For many of us, drinking was a way to silence the voice. Maybe it's telling us, *This marriage isn't working*, but an evening martini helps us stay another day. It could be telling us *I need to make changes in my life*, but we are scared, so we have a few afternoon beers in the sun and the voice goes quiet.

But it always returns.

For Amanda, the voice told her to stop drinking. Although none of her friends or her husband thought she had a problem, Amanda knew. Her father drank throughout her childhood, and from her first Bartles & Jaymes wine cooler at age fourteen, Amanda had a dysfunctional relationship with booze. She blacked out for the first time at sixteen. She began to understand that when her friends said they "passed out," it was not the same as what happened to Amanda, which was that she was awake and speaking with people—sometimes for hours—but would have no memory of these hours the following morning. None. She would remember talking, or a dim room, and then blackness. The dread that engulfed her after a night of heavy drinking was pure anguish. She took online quizzes titled "Are You An Alcoholic?" (The answer was usually *Maybe, maybe not.*)

Amanda told herself that if she were not yet an alcoholic, she did not have to stop drinking. And so she did not stop. Amanda drank through college, through years of travel in Greece, Egypt, Kenya, and Europe. She wrote about drinking. She fell in love many times, and then she really fell in love. She married, had children, published novels. To absolutely everyone, she was fine.

Her true heart told her, *You are not fine.*

She felt uneasy. She stopped drinking as a test run, started again. She convinced herself she was not like the people in the AA meetings she attended—any meeting she went to, she found a way to distinguish herself from them—*I'm younger than everyone in this meeting; I'm employed and that lady just got fired; I'm more put together than that guy; I'm older and more experienced than all the kids in this meeting.* (Although when someone spoke at these meetings, it was as if they knew her brain better than anyone in her "real" life.) She drank good wine, fancy cocktails; she was *fun*! But ignoring her heart was taking a toll. Life with small children was hard. To keep up, to work and play and be the mom and wife she thought she was supposed to be, she drank. Wine enabled her to pack lunches, to read another story at bedtime, to stand in front of large audiences in a fancy outfit and speak about literature though she was exhausted and scared.

(The heroines of Amanda's books were often scared. Amanda's true heart spoke through her fictional characters.)

Now, Amanda looks back and mourns the years she wasted trying desperately to keep wine in her life. She was so ashamed every time she overdid it, so disappointed in herself. She tells herself that she needed to feel all this despair to get to where she is now, understanding without a doubt that her life is better sober. Dwelling on the regrets is wasted energy, she tells herself, and sometimes she listens. The shame, for Amanda, has been slowly but surely replaced with radiant pride.

On New Year's Day, after a New Year's Eve blackout, Amanda vowed she would never overdo it again. A few months later, after a speaking engagement that she had been honored to receive, she blacked out.

On Easter morning, Amanda dressed her beautiful children in perfect outfits. She went to a glamorous friend's house, and the mothers drank pink prosecco while they hid Easter eggs. An idyllic day. Everything's great, life is grand!

She woke at 3:00 a.m. on the couch in her home, still wearing her silk Easter dress. She remembered the Easter brisket, braided Easter bread. She remembered going to another friend's house and watching her kids jump on a trampoline, while she sipped red wine. Then nothing.

Lying on her couch at 3:00 a.m., the doom enveloped Amanda, and as usual, her true heart spoke.

It said, *This is not your life.*

For the first time, and crying, Amanda listened.

This was her Day One.

CONSCIOUSNESS
EXPERIMENTS

✴

But when the world is, indeed, in chaos,
then an affirmation of cosmos becomes essential.

~MADELEINE L'ENGLE

MILES DAVIS + CEDAR SMOKE

REVOLUTION

LUCID DREAMING

PSYCHEDELIC LUNCH

BATHING IN SOUND

VOLUNTEERING

ZERO-GRAVITY FLOAT TANK

TEA LEAVES, TIGERS + TAROT

MILES DAVIS + CEDAR SMOKE

ncense is a way to connect to another plane of experience—to the olfactory dimension. Sometimes we lose touch with that sense, and then, just by holding a thin little stick to the stove's flame, we wake up a big part of our soul.

Jardine is a fiend for incense, having fallen in love immediately with the starter incense she bought as a teenager at a head shop on Cape Cod, and graduating to all kinds of Japanese, Indian, and French stuff. There are no rules to incense—you sometimes find the transcendent ones in cheap boxes on the tables of street vendors, or mistakenly buy boxes in high-end boutiques that are too vanilla or fake-floral. So you get to enjoy the thrill of the hunt, sniffing and burning, letting some other part beside your brain decide. It's such a good feeling to activate various faculties in your own consciousness, and even to treat it as a game. In our society, the intellect is overrated. Why not dream with some other side of our self?

Before we got sober, we didn't necessarily like messing around with consciousness because, to be honest, our poor dear little nervous systems were often fragile and bruised, and we just felt like surviving the hour was good enough. Now we more frequently feel a plush awareness, or a luxury of awakeness—we have more room to play.

Having a spectrum of incenses also lets you mark different times in your day, or seasons in your life. There's a fig incense that transports Jardine immediately back to graduate school in Ann Arbor, Michigan, to an attic apartment with slanted ceilings and a lot of sunlight. A box of mesquite cones she bought in Marfa, Texas, reminds her of rusted fences, falcons, and infinite clouds. And almost every morning these days, she starts with dark coffee, cedar incense, and Miles Davis—this is her sturdy little bridge into work mode.

Incense can offer an anchor to the complexity of an hour, or another passageway into the moment. It helps to silently and powerfully mark time. Its smoke slowly twists off the tiny red cinder on the tip of the stick, reminding us that nothing lasts, that heat is ephemeral, that everything changes form, and that this is beautiful.

REVOLUTION

There's nothing like a drunk dinner table talking politics. People can get red-faced, sweaty, the issues heating up the room like a furnace. And this isn't by nature bad, or useless—people can become clearer in their convictions or change points of view, and bond during these debates.

As life in the United States has gone haywire recently too, many Americans also talk about drinking *away* the daily news. And for some people, that will work, and it won't hinder them from still making change or protesting.

But for us, drinking and being politically or socially active didn't quite fit together. It was when we subtracted liquor and drugs that there was space for marching, for volunteering, for joining.

It was funny for Jardine to watch her mind go bonkers with a particular kind of über-self-conscious thinking that has always affected her: *If I go to this march tomorrow, will I look self-righteous? If I volunteer to teach at the prison, will it look like I think I'm a savior, a martyr, that I know more than the incarcerated women? If I don't fully understand all facets of the issue, and I've always been confused about this particular legislation, is it fair of me to join this protest? Am I an imposter, a wannabe?*

Sobriety has given Jardine a tolerance and patience for her own mixed emotions, a kindness to herself, that lets her go forward in earnest without caring how it looks. In a parallel way, one of the original problems she had in getting sober was fearing people would think that she thought it was a "superior" thing to do. She certainly doesn't think that, and most people probably don't even notice what she's up to in this regard, all of which is beside the point because WHO CARES?

Jardine realized that her personal agenda in volunteering and marching and donating would always be complex, with elements in there of needing validation, wanting to be seen as good, craving a place in a strong movement. And these desires coexist with a desire to give forward what she's been given in her life, to connect with other human beings, to stand up for what she believes is right, and to join forces so she can be enlightened and educated and motivated.

LUCID DREAMING

Amanda didn't used to remember her dreams, and believed she didn't dream at all. She had read that alcohol increases the number of times you wake in the night (when its sedating effect wears off), and many sober friends had told her about the newfound joy of deep, real sleep, so she was excited to explore the underworld of her awareness now that she was sober and uncompromised.

Amanda read about lucid dreaming, about training herself to be aware she was dreaming *inside* her dreams. Some people claim they can control their dreams, even harness that brainpower to enhance creativity. Dreams can be the ultimate meditation, where you try out life choices before committing, deeply process creative questions in work and play, and overcome anxiety by testing scary situations in a safe zone.

Where else but in a dream can you be a virtuoso violinist if you've never picked up an instrument? We fly to Mars, swim in the sea, lunch with loved ones who have passed on, or hang out with

Shakespeare. And we love—beholden to no laws, moral or otherwise.

There's a history of people controlling dreams, from the Ancient Greeks and Tibetan monks, to Marquis d'Hervey de Saint-Denys, who wrote books about nocturnal magic and sprinkled women's signature perfumes on his pillowcase to see how scents affected his dream narratives. Gurus offer dream workshops in Hawaii and the Netherlands and Seoul and Arizona. Amanda wants to find a pot of gold so she can attend . . . hey, a girl can dream!

Although in her research Amanda found recommendations for supplements like Galantamine, she refrained. Some dreaming aficionados swoon for sleep headsets that detect REM sleep and deliver flashing light cues that a dreamer can pick up on, therefore knowing they are dreaming. A Luddite at heart, Amanda began with a dream journal by her bedside. But she felt she needed more guidance.

Even though she was scared of her subconscious, memories, and dreams, Amanda tracked down an online course for lucid dreaming. The website gave her two options: "YES, take the online course," or "NO, I want my mind to remain locked." Well! A locked mind is no one's idea of a good time, so Amanda signed up. And thus her free e-mail workshop began.

Amanda's kids were very interested in her project. Her eldest son claimed he never dreamed either. Her youngest daughter (aged seven) said that *obviously* you could control your dreams—she'd done it "literally millions of times." When pressed for details, she said, "I change the channel if something bad is happening" or "just open a door in the sky if I'm scared and Mom, like, pops out and hugs me."

On night one, Amanda was instructed to say to her pillow, "I will remember my dreams" three times. On her night table, she placed a ballpoint pen and her journal, which she left opened to a blank page to be filled in the next morning with the date and a dream title (and drew a box for any illustrations). She tried to notice her body falling asleep, and then she fell asleep. But when she woke up and gave herself a few minutes to recapture her nighttime adventures, she remembered . . . nothing.

Amanda was supposed to lie still for five minutes, trying to remember, before picking up her phone or getting out of bed. The minutes ticked by, but there was still nothing.

Over morning donuts, Amanda's daughter announced she'd dreamed of running into an alligator on a hiking trail, wrestling with it, and emerging victorious. Amanda's husband had a nightmare about being unable to fill out health insurance forms.

That day, as instructed by her dream guru, Amanda asked herself if she was dreaming or if she was awake twenty to thirty times. Then she performed a "reality check" by looking in a mirror (because the word is that reflections in dreams don't work correctly); flipping a light switch on and off (apparently, you can't control light in dreams); trying to push her fingers through a solid object (only works in dreams); or staring at her hands (in real life, your hand looks like a hand, whereas in dreams, it might look strange or have a weird number of fingers).

Amanda found that even asking herself if she was dreaming made her world a bit trippy. The low, evening light over Barton Springs, making her children gleam in the water: Was Amanda really sure she wasn't dreaming? She pressed into the grass, which held up: not dreaming. During her dog walk, as she heard cicadas and felt the Austin heat, Amanda wondered, *Am I dreaming?* Is that *my* mini schnauzer or a *dream* mini schnauzer? She tried to push one hand through the other. Nope.

That night, Amanda readied her dream notebook. Then she closed her eyes and focused on the morphing shapes behind her eyelids. She fell asleep. In the morning, she heard her mini schnauzer barking and opened her eyes. As instructed, she tried for a millisecond to remember her dreams. *I don't remember my*— she thought, but then realized she *did* remember some things. For the first time in her entire life, Amanda reentered her dreamscape, hurriedly jotting it all down: houses she'd been in, a weird scenario about her aunt knitting a poncho, a pile of jigsaw puzzles waiting to be solved.

She had dreamed! It felt like breaking through to new knowledge. Amanda had been too frightened to allow herself to know her dreams. But now she was safe—she was ready. Dreaming about her aunt's soft maroon poncho didn't seem so scary, in the end. It was wondrous.

And the places she'd traveled in this first remembered dream felt familiar. She'd been in these houses before but couldn't remember anywhere in her waking life that resembled them. Were they homes she'd visited as a child? Or places she'd constructed in her dreams? Or were they places she'd just conjured the night before but her dreams made them feel familiar? Was she dreaming now? (She looked at her hand, but it just looked like a hand.)

So much lay ahead: harnessing her dreams for creativity, exploring how to wake within her dreams. Amanda ordered a hardcover book about dreams that also had blank pages for writing what she remembered and illustrations to help interpret dream images.

But what felt revelatory was that she wasn't learning to remember her dreams for her kids, for her husband, or for anyone else. There was no monetary value to this work, no burning need for it. Amanda was taking the time to consider herself, to deem her visions worthy of care and investment. Maybe that was the dream.

PSYCHEDELIC LUNCH

Jardine met an artist who had just moved onto her block in Austin—Jardine lived "up the hill" and Denise Prince lived "down the hill," and they quickly saw something in each other, a spark of mischief, or a head full of esoteric questions that would make most people roll their eyes, and both were wary but wondered about the other.

For Jardine, as for many human beings, any social interaction is slightly awkward, and her instinct is to avoid them entirely. Even when she looks forward to a social event, she drags her feet, makes up excuses not to go, for no reason. One of her favorite ideas to fall back on these days, to escape real engagement, is that people don't make friends after a certain age, and she'd reached that age. But Denise invited Jardine for lunch one day, so Jardine went down the hill.

Jardine knocked on the door and was breathless when she walked inside. Denise had closed the curtains, lit jewellike lamps and candles, and set the table with antique plates. Denise had a standard poodle named Mister Darcy, and he was gigantic and yet able to romp around in delicate and elegant circles. His hair was curled and shining like black licorice, and he barely fit into the house.

There was a regal whiff to this ordinary day, like Denise picked an hour and put a crown on it and made it the queen. She poured two-dollar rosewater she'd gotten at a Turkish grocery and Topo Chico into gold-etched glasses. Put a record on her tiny toy record player, and they sat down to a simple lunch of salmon with green herbs and ginger sauce and a salad. Then she brought out hot tea on a tray, and little ice creams with a cookie on the side.

They talked, opening up, unraveling, spilling, dreaming. The records—Jardine wishes she could remember—bounced from kids' music to garage rock to classical piano.

Let's just say that when Jardine walked back into the Texas sunshine, she was tripping on life. They've since become best friends, worked on projects together, helped each other dream new dreams, and fully loved saying "come up the hill for tea" or "come down the hill for a bite" because it made Austin into the English countryside of 1905. Screw all that mumbo-jumbo about being set; we want to make new friends over psychedelic lunches until we die.

Amanda, who works like hell while her kids are at school and wants only to be with them afterward, makes time for such lunches *out*. Her favorite spot is an Italian restaurant called Juliet about four minutes from her house. She invites a writer she admires or a friend she misses, and they twirl spaghetti Bolognese and laugh and sometimes order the spumoni sundae for dessert. It would be easy to sit back and say she's too busy or can't even afford the lunchtime special menu, but giving up on new people or enchanting interruptions of daily life is dangerous. Motherhood, the writing life, *and* sobriety can be isolating, even for her introverted self. Jardine and Amanda were at one point these new friends to each other, stealing an hour to take a summer walk around the lake, grabbing an iced coffee, then going back to the routine. They are extremely grateful they took the time.

So why not invite a new acquaintance to watercress sandwiches and oolong tea, put some sidewalk daisies in a vase, and listen to records: Françoise Hardy, La Femme, Jefferson Airplane? Do it in the middle of the workday, then race back to whatever you were doing and relish the strange taste in your mouth, the distortion to your environment, and sense of what—and who—is possible.

BATHING IN SOUND

New to Los Angeles, Jardine heard the term *sound bath* a lot but didn't know what it was, and here in California, everyone was doing it, or having it done, or advertising it, or reminiscing about their latest sound bath. She was determined to learn.

Turns out a sound bath is what you might imagine: you get washed by bells and harps and drums. It's like an invisible spirit pours music delicately through your mind, immersing your heart in it, rinsing your organs. It's one of those experiences that goes through you.

Jardine and her partner, Neil, signed up for a sound-bath evening session at the yoga center down the block. The happily crowded space had Friday-night energy, an air of anticipation, a sense of sexuality and sparks, as people arranged mats that touched at the edges. It was summer and the door was open to the street. The instructors sat on the floor at the front, instruments set up on either side, and led the group in chanting and meditation, then told them to lie down and get comfortable.

Once everyone closed their eyes, the instructors played the instruments in a way that flowed over us all, and the street noise came in and was married to the sound bath. Sirens, laughter, a bottle breaking, braided into the harp, the drum, the lute. It was better that way, the practice connected to the Los Angeles neighborhood after dark, because everyone lying down and listening didn't have to choose between real and unreal, inside or outside, us or them. It was all one piece.

Even though no one physically touched her, Jardine felt spoiled and coddled. Like someone was using a gold comb on her emotions, gently raking them. Softening them, curling them up with a sweet hand.

A variation on this idea, useful when there's no time for the yoga center, is digital soundscapes and—most important—binaural beats. Jardine has embraced the concept of binaural beats, without having any idea what on earth they really are or how they work. She regularly plugs her headphones into her laptop and goes to a sound engineer's website offering dozens of configurations of natural sounds and binaural beats. The beats supposedly reach or stimulate different parts of the brain. Focus, creativity, sleep—there's a binaural-beat equation for each. She loves this little noise library, and always feels like someone out of *Blade Runner* or *Neuromancer,* listening to the future.

VOLUNTEERING

Asober friend volunteers for Meals on Wheels and loves the simplicity of bringing someone food—it's an ancient ritual, in a sense. Delivering food to her neighbors takes her out of her head, introduces her to her own community (which is almost rare in this modern world), helps her consistently recognize how lucky she is and have respect for how difficult life can be, and gives her warmth and connection in the exchange. And a hungry soul gets a hot dinner.

That friend loves counting on this regular appointment, but if we can't commit to a weekly or monthly gig, we can volunteer for a one-off event. Another friend always works on an annual party to support the local women's shelter, calling on friends to cooperatively build stands and tents and donate time and food and toys.

Jardine doesn't have kids and has an offbeat freelance schedule, and while she'd volunteered here and there in the past, sobriety meant she had more time and more bandwidth. So she volunteered for a "personal storytelling" program in a Texas prison. She could write a book on what she learned from the incarcerated women in those workshops, how they taught her about strength, humanity, our justice system, beauty, our class hierarchy, violence, loss, love, regret; the conversations and stories transcended the cold sterile locked rooms. What she didn't expect to affect her so deeply was carpooling with the other volunteers—an hour ride each way that, over the course of a few years, changed her life.

The prison program was founded eighteen years previously by two openhearted women who used tools from a more hippie, intuitive, feminist culture than the slightly puritanical or patriarchal and academic one Jardine came from. Every carpooler had to "share" for two minutes, speaking uninterrupted about her mood and thoughts (good or bad), and what was going on in her life. The other women listened without judgment.

There was no room to fix each other, and this "holding space for each other" and zero-preaching attitude was the core of the prison workshop as well. Candor and mutual respect are also at the foundation for 12-step programs, which pivot on sharing stories, listening without judgment, and creating space for diverse and even contradictory experiences. No leader. No authority figure in the room.

The age of the women in the carpool spanned forty years, and while Jardine started out skeptical of this new style of communicating and bonding, she was amazed by the rewards. To listen can be healing and affirmative, and so can being heard.

The volunteers all shared on the way home; it was night, and they'd been at the prison for hours, heard stuff that broke their hearts or enlightened them. Jardine listened intently as these women, once strangers to her, each one coming from a different world, religion, and generation, spoke about fears and beautiful observations and insecurities for two minutes at a time.

Jardine watched out the back-seat window as the highway, farm fences, and yucca plants were silhouetted against a burning-blue horizon, the stars and moon hanging in the black velvet sky above them, and she thought, *Teachers are everywhere, wisdom is everywhere.*

ZERO-GRAVITY FLOAT TANK

Otherwise known as sensory-deprivation tanks, or isolation chambers, float tanks offer a sort of "organic tripping." This is freedom, this is dreamtime, this is an experiment you can build into the lunch hour of an average workday and blow your sense of reality to beautiful shreds. (As you've probably noticed by now, we sometimes love to nurture our sense of order and comprehension, and, quite often, we love to ruin it!)

A float tank is basically a chamber or pod that can be closed so no light or sound gets in. The body-temperature water is knee-deep but so full of salt that we float no matter what; the air is kept at the same exact temperature as the water so we can't tell where water and air meet, and where our bodies and selves begin and end. There's no stimulation, from any direction, no need to maintain physical vigilance or coordination. Our bodies fully relax and we sink into reverie or mediation or hallucination easily while hovering—weightless—in the hour.

When Jardine was little, she played in tide pools made by sandbars between the ocean and shore. They were separate from the main body of water—and finite, just lasting an hour sometimes while the landscape shifted—and so their water warmed up like a bathtub. She'd loll about in these giant puddles, chase tiny translucent fish, hold up seaweed and shake it at a little brother like she was the monster. Float tanks remind her of these memories, buoyed between waking and dreaming.

To feel no gravity, to be set free of that earthly condition, is a pleasure. But it can also be scary. She's had instances of succumbing to the dark but somehow getting jolted into fear. She suddenly didn't want to be alone with her mind, and it took a minute to ease into the extreme solitude. It helped that pounds and pounds of dissolved salt healed her as she drifted, and a clean robe hung outside the pod for when she was done.

So close your eyes, and breathe. Let the psychedelic visions play out, if you want, in your head. Compose a poem or a bit of music. Meditate. Talk to yourself. Have an epiphany. We can leave the door propped open if we're claustrophobic. Or we can leave. If there's something we know for sure by now, one lady's vision quest is another man's nightmare. Find your way, little fish.

It can feel like science fiction behind the pod's metal door. The body floats, pressed to the surface like it's called up. We're stars, rotating in the dark, full of energy and light, hanging in a different kind of sky. What happens comes from the magic of physics and brain chemistry, the supernatural workings of earthly minds.

When the glowing blue light slowly comes back, we emerge from the chamber, shower off the salt and the visions, and wear a fluffy robe to the lounge. Coloring books and sketch pads are there and we sip chamomile tea and listen to space-age music and doodle or write down bits of ideas or nonsense. When we finally get dressed and leave the little storefront in the strip mall, we take with us nets of caught memories, an incandescence around our head like a veil. We belong to the underworld and the overworld, our heart working in slow motion.

TEA LEAVES, TIGERS + TAROT

O h, we have questions. So many questions. And when we stop smothering them, the questions get loud: *Will I end up alone? Are my loved ones safe? Will all my dreams come true? Come to think of it, what* are *all my dreams?*

We've always loved this advice from Rainer Maria Rilke: "Be patient toward all that is unsolved in your heart and try to love the questions themselves, like locked rooms and like books that are now written in a very foreign tongue. Do not now seek to know the answers, which cannot be given you because you would not be able to live them. And the point is, to live everything."

I Ching, tea leaves, palm reading. Tarot. These are ways of accessing divine clues, especially if they're not practiced as literal fortune-telling tools. They offer a method of sitting with the unknown in an organized way, with someone by our side. The mission for us is as much exploring as discovering, as much wondering as knowing. Which doesn't mean we don't crave the solution, the facts, the prognosis. We're just learning, slowly, with love, by the wisdom of others, to live in the absence of the definite.

Amanda researched tarot but balked at having her own cards read. She didn't believe in tarot cards! And also, she believed too much. What if the reader told her something terrible would happen? She was afraid. But smart friends insisted a tarot reading was not a prediction but a way to reflect on herself.

Come to think of it, reflecting on herself sounded *more* terrifying. But one purpose of writing *The Sober Lush* was to inspire others to be brave, so in solidarity (and so as not to be a sober hypocrite), Amanda decided to give tarot a shot, and made an appointment online. Her fears were not allayed by a confirmation e-mail instructing her to park outside a "big witchy raw cedar fence." She was instructed to open "an elaborate gate with a dragon door pull," enter a yard, and look for the "cute vintage Royal Spartanette trailer." The tarot reader wrote, "I'll be inside the trailer waiting for you."

Yikes!

On the day of her reading, Amanda found herself paralyzed outside the witchy fence. She texted Jardine, who said she couldn't wait to hear about the session. Amanda considered driving home to hide under the covers and maybe eat some Junior Mints.

She got out of her dented Mazda 5. The dragon door glinted in the late-afternoon sun. She opened the gate and walked past a house and toward a trailer.

"Hi, love!" called the tarot reader, Angeliska, of Sister Temperance Tarot.

Angeliska's greeting was disarmingly cheerful. Amanda went inside the trailer and was offered a drink, a seat. Amanda asked to use the restroom, and Angeliska said gently there was no restroom and if Amanda had carefully read the confirmation e-mail (and/or answered the phone when Angeliska called to go over the confirmation e-mail), Amanda would have known there was no restroom.

"Oh, I'll be fine," said Amanda. Rather than feeling ashamed for having disappointed Angeliska (Amanda *had* speed-read the confirmation e-mail), Amanda did feel fine, so something good was happening. The candlelit trailer was perfumed with thick incense smoke. Amanda turned on her phone to record audio.

Angeliska sat back and asked, "What do you want to focus on today?"

"I don't know," said Amanda. Her questions were so all pervasive that it seemed impossible to focus on one.

"What's going on in your world?" asked Angeliska. Her eyes were large, glittering with eye shadow. Her smile was genuine and welcoming. Amanda exhaled and began to speak. She talked about work, love, and fear.

Angeliska laid out nine cards, then added six more as they spoke. The session felt like an hour with a brilliant therapist. When Amanda later replayed the audio recording, she could hear Angeliska pointing and referring to cards, but during the hour, it had felt as if Angeliska were just listening. As if Amanda had a supercool older sister who wore gold eye shadow and genuinely *heard* Amanda.

Amanda struggles with the past, said Angeliska (the Six of Swords—a woman and child being rowed across turbulent water in a boat filled with swords, which Angeliska said could represent emotional baggage). She needs to purge her metaphorical rowboat and move on.

Amanda, said Angeliska, is afraid of joy. She needs to get quiet with herself. She has an incredible group of women around her (Three of Cups—an illustration of three beautiful women in togas raising goblets, perhaps filled with fizzy water instead of wine). She needs to get naked more (the Two of Cups, showing two lovers) and recognize the love she has (the Ten of Cups, depicting a couple and their children under a rainbow).

And in the center: the Seven of Wands, a "warrior playing whack-a-mole." Angeliska pointed out that Amanda is in a constant state of preparing for battle. "When the tiger is there," said Angeliska, "you can deal with it. But always worrying, *Is there a tiger?* That isn't useful."

Amanda said, "Wow." Her brain said, *Is there a tiger?*

"Worrying is praying for things you don't want to happen," said Angeliska.

"Whoa," said Amanda. Her brain said, *Is there a tiger? Because I'm ready, if so.*

"To retrain yourself out of that mind-set is going to be a big thing, I think," said Angeliska.

Amanda nodded. Her brain said—well, you get the picture.

As Angeliska spoke, Amanda felt hot, dizzy. She blinked back tears and felt understood. Angeliska didn't answer any of Amanda's questions directly. She told her, "The most accurate way to know the future is to create it." Amanda realized she sort of wanted concrete answers but would have been skeptical if she had been given them.

Instead, she sat in the trailer that had no restroom as a tiny bell was rung. Amanda then felt the warmth of Angeliska's hands as she wrapped them around her own hands. Angeliska was thanking the mysterious universe, but Amanda wasn't listening to her words.

This is what Amanda heard: "You've made it this far. You've survived a lot. The questions will continue to come, and you're strong enough to hear them." And, as Angeliska said, when they hugged her goodbye, "Text me anytime. Hey. Listen. You're not alone."

PLAYING

The most sophisticated people I know—
inside they are all children.

~JIM HENSON

SECRET ROPE SWING

ROLLER SKATES

DO YOU WANNA DANCE?

THE BEST DEFENSE IS A GOOD OFFENSE

CLIMBING ROCKS

GLITTERING FERRIS WHEEL

KARAOKE

FORMULA 1

DONKEY KONG + RED BULL

SECRET ROPE SWING

n high school, Jardine's friends sneaked out during the spring months to a secret rope swing near a lake. It was technically on the property of a stranger's summerhouse, but no one ever saw them, and trespassing added to the fun. The swing was a knotted hempy line hanging from a tree over blue water, right out of Tom Sawyer's world, and kids ecstatically pushed one another off the ledge.

They'd bring Camel Lights and a boom box with a Blondie tape or Grateful Dead bootleg, and lose track of hours within seconds. The cold, mysterious, deep, dark water was rimmed by grass and wildflowers. Both boys and girls flocked to the rope. They rarely wore bathing suits, swimming instead in cutoff corduroys and T-shirts, because the swing was usually a spontaneous decision.

Except for one night, when they wore nothing. And if trespassing during the day was bad and forbidden, rope-swinging at night and *naked* was a cardinal sin. Looking back, it was outrageously innocent. To this day she can't remember who suggested it, but it seemed inevitable—it was going to happen. Jardine remembers waiting in an antsy line of maybe five skinny-dipping swimmers—the woods were so dark that everyone was just a possibility; no one was a body. The giggling and nervous bad jokes stole through the chamber of space among the trees, and they made dust with their bare feet.

Her turn—she stepped up, got warned to release the rope carefully by someone who had *not* and thus chafed their inner thighs, and she took a moment to consider the big emptiness. Reflections of stars glimmered on the slick black surface. Then she pushed off, floated in the air, and finally let go, was somehow suspended in the sky, then she was falling and falling and falling; she splashed (immersed, vanished, hidden) and finally burst up in a froth of icy water, laughing and gasping for breath.

The water in that moment knew every secret she'd ever had, and loved her more for it.

How is that? How is it that skinny-dipping can mean the meager difference between nothing at all and just a few inches of bikini or bathing shorts, yet the feeling of being naked in the water is so much more exhilarating? Of course, it's due to feeling—consciously or subconsciously—like we're breaking a rule.

But it also feels like tapping into pure pleasure, like garden-of-Eden stuff, ancient possibilities. Naked is how we came into this world, and most of us have been "dressed" ever since, so sunbathing nude in a backyard, the shadows of an elm tree moving over your skin, the sun warming your whole body, is a way to shed social niceties, remove the burden of "should" and "have to." Just walking around the house for an hour or so in our birthday suit reminds us we're physical, we exist as bodies, and we're not just a chaos of thought and emotion above our shoulders. Some of us, ahem, benefit from that reminder.

Skinny-dipping and sunbathing in the nude can mean titillation to one person and radical self-acceptance to another. It can mean animalistic relaxation, like when cats lie in the afternoon light for hours. Or it can mean all those things. Jardine knows a couple, mischievous and young at heart, who were always vague about their vacations. Because they went to nudist colonies and kept their adventures to themselves. She finally got them to spill about a new international naked-communes-and-hotels network they discovered made of cool and progressive spots around the world. She promised not to tell, but you can find out by asking around and investigating online.

Jardine went to a Korean bathhouse recently, a four-story village of hedonism and humanity in the middle of Los Angeles. Women of all shapes and sizes and ages and backgrounds walked around the women's floor naked, dipped into pools and saunas, taking care of themselves, floating, showering, thinking. Twenty languages could be heard as people laughed and chatted with a friend or mother or sister or daughter. Jardine was alone but not alone. She went from being hyper-self-conscious (in fact, self-conscious of her self-consciousness) to letting go as she watched other women let go. She sat in a heated pool, arms out on the cool tile, and her face turned red and her heartbeat slowed. A woman—older than her, black hair piled in a beautiful topknot—gestured to Jardine (since they didn't speak the same language) that it was time to revive herself in the ice bath. So Jardine went, her face contorted as she submerged her body into the chill, and her blood pumped like a drumbeat. She breathed fast, so alive. Then the woman grinned—wearing bright red lipstick in the pool, superglam—and waved to Jardine to come back to the hot pool. And so she did.

ROLLER SKATES

Amanda was once eleven years old in roller skates, racing her sisters down the street. She moved fast, taking for granted her strength and invincibility. She skated backward, hair whirling, a boom box playing Madonna and INXS. She fell and rose again; the shadows lengthening, the streetlights flashing on. The streets at night were her disco, her playground, until her mother called Amanda and her sisters home.

Somehow, over the years, we became the ones who nursed whiskey and watched others dance. We raised our eyebrows at goofballs; when a voice inside said, *Get up and join in*, we shut the voice down with another drink. We became inhibited, afraid of letting go. We almost forgot how to play for the joy of playing. We avoided any chance of becoming objects of ridicule.

When she first got sober, Amanda realized that she no longer knew how to have fun.

She remembered how much she loved roller skating. When her children asked her—for the hundredth time—to join them at the roller rink, she surprised them by saying yes. The skates were strange on her feet. She buckled and crumpled like a foal. A voice in her mind told her she was making a fool of herself as she lurched around the rink.

At Playland Skate Park in Austin, there are Saturday Races. When it was time for the "Women Over Eighteen" category, she bit her lip. Her son said, "Come on, Mom, go!" She made her way, shakily, to the starting line.

As she raced, she remembered her purple leg warmers. How sleek she'd felt in them, zooming down the street. She was still that girl, the fastest girl in the neighborhood, the one with two French braids. A rediscovered road ribboned before her: drawing, singing, making things from clay, telling absurd jokes, laughing at absurd jokes, roller skating. That girl had been waiting to come back out to play.

The race ended long before she crossed the finish line. She hadn't won, but then again, she had won.

DO YOU WANNA DANCE?

s there anything as magnanimous as a dance floor? Everyone is welcome. Bass beat thunders through our rib cages, lights falling like raindrops in the big bad room, other dancers letting go and being alive all around us, with us, touching us, disappearing and reappearing; nothing is solid. To be quite frank, we often say *no thanks* to dancing invitations because we don't feel like getting to the club, or staying up that late, or making the transition from daylight person to wild child. But holy hell, is it good for us when we do.

Dancing feels like pure id, the ego left at the door, the core of us set free. We think Daybreaker and Ecstatic Dance and other "conscious raves" are genius, and we love the celebration and liberty and sequins in their sober spirits. Why not wake up with some yoga and a mob of happy dancing souls? Daybreaker alone is in cities across the world now, and the idea is contagious.

Starting the day with such raw frenzy and playtime is about throwing off the constricting suit of our self-consciousness and pride. Put on some zebra pajamas and rainbow unicorn horns and gold lipstick instead. That this sort of festivity exists makes us happy—it's evidence dancing doesn't belong exclusively to drugs and alcohol.

When we first stopped drinking, one of the most comfortable nightlife options in Austin, Texas, was two-stepping at dance halls such as the Broken Spoke. People drank there, but it wasn't why we showed up—we came to dance. Cowboys and cowgirls, pink-cheeked young folks, white-braided gentlemen, novices and old-schoolers— we all danced. The formal way a person would invite us to dance at the beginning of a song, and the way we would go out onto the floor, and take each other's hands—sometimes that added up to more connection by the time the band wound down the tune than we had in the course of a whole mad crazy bender. After, everyone would drift into the parking lot, stand against vintage cars, and smoke, and talk, and we always felt very shy and very, very real.

THE BEST DEFENSE
IS A GOOD OFFENSE

One of the reasons Jardine feels lucky to have been born in her generation was that for her mother's generation, competitive girls' sports were barely an option. Jardine never considered herself an athlete, and yet the things she took away from years of being on teams are still with her, from holding your own, to relying on others, to not hogging the ball, to realizing there is no victory unless it's a group victory, to shaking hands even when you lose.

Her favorite sport was ice hockey, not *despite* how bad she was at it but maybe *because* she was so bad. Falling down was part of every practice, every game. Her team even had drills where the players had to sprint and fall, get up, sprint and fall. They wore shoulder and knee pads that smelled like rotting cabbage, and they blew snot down their jerseys. There was no choice but to check the ego and abandon any social obligation to smell good, be sweet, or look pretty when they went over the boards and onto the ice. It was awesome.

Amanda also played high school (and college) ice hockey, and remembers the ferocity and thrill of listening to "Welcome to the Jungle" and "Paradise City" by Guns N' Roses in the locker room before bursting onto the ice. In a funny parallel, this blissfully maniacal warrior mode reminds us of how we often felt at dive bars, dancing and sweating to the jukebox, and roughhousing with friends, spilling beer on ourselves, being raunchy, nasty, impolite.

These days, a few of our friends have joined soccer leagues or play club volleyball. Getting on a field or court lets us slip the straightjacket of social niceties, get the camaraderie of a locker room, and touch base with the sense that nothing matters except what's happening precisely at that moment. Sports are myopic by nature, and tunnel vision can be a really welcome break from family affairs and work crises and LIFE in general. There's just a tennis ball, a racket, a net, an opponent, and a very carefully delineated *in* and *out*.

We also dig fitness classes because people collectively drop the veneer. Everyone's vulnerable, sweaty, messy, and there's a good vibe when we walk out and slug water and wipe faces with towels. We love that for an hour we put our life into an instructor's hands. This is an ongoing idea in a lot of our new practices, this desire to take the phone off the hook. To let someone tell us to do it faster, keep going, stand up and sit down; they play Missy Elliott at volume 11; they are the cheerleader to our quarterback.

The sports and fitness outlet for sober people sometimes ends in a seesaw syndrome though. We've seen friends quit drinking *and* go carb free *and* begin a mega-training program, all on the same day. We get it—we want to be better, to be powerful, *now*. (And many do lose weight after quitting drinking. Faces get brighter, hair and nails stronger. Before and After pictures are common on sober social media.) But it's also okay (and maybe better?) to take it step by step. If the endeavor is too exhausting, everything is eventually abandoned in one day, just as it began. For us, we've found that relentlessly diabolically masochistically aiming for an idealized body isn't as fun as swimming and biking and stretching and walking on a whim and maybe even dancing with our daughter while we sob dramatically to Taylor Swift's "Back to December" in our pajamas for the hell of it.

CLIMBING ROCKS

Jardine started hiking the Barton Creek Greenbelt in Austin by herself when she got sober. But she wasn't actually alone: at one juncture in the trail, if you look up through the brush to the limestone cliffs, you'll always catch impressions of movement—bare backs, rope, tattoos. She was never sure what those people were doing. But she was curious, because they seemed like a tribe, and she assumed all tribes were closed.

She had recently forgone Austin's dive-bar scene to discover what went on in the daylight. But so far she was just lonely, having given up one world without locating the next.

It was by pure chance that a year later she started dating one of these tribesmen—a rock climber who would come home, hands battered with cuts and sticky with chalk dust like powdered sugar, practically high from climbing. He told her that women are natural climbers because they tend to use their legs rather than their arms for strength, and they're typically more nimble. He wore her down enough to buy climbing shoes—hard-rubber things like ballet toe shoes—and lured her to those cliffs she'd seen.

At the site, she received tutorials on teamwork (she would clip into a safety rope that a partner on the ground held in case she fell) and technique (use your core, be patient, say "Falling!" before you fall). Then she stepped up to the wall of stone. It was a funny moment, her first confrontation with the rock. She felt like someone was asking her a question, and she couldn't even fathom what language they were speaking, let alone come up with an answer.

But she did ultimately learn this: there's a lot to be said for starting something you don't know how to finish, something you can't fully control. Climbing for her was not just shaking hands with fear but pressing her whole body against it. Midway up, she was hanging in the sky, legs quaking with fatigue and anxiety, a condition that climbers call "the Elvis shakes." Once climbing, it's easy to rush each move, as if pursued by vulnerability itself, but it's an invaluable experience to stop, quiet the mind, and look at the situation. Each time she did that, she would suddenly see a way that had been invisible, a viable combination of handgrips and footholds that she could use. Her muscles felt depleted as she reached for the top. But the strangers below, standing in sunshine filtering through the tall trees—people she'd skeptically eyed months before when she hiked past—cheered her on as she pulled herself over the rock's sharp lip.

On the way up, she'd avoided looking down, too terrified to see how far she could fall. But now, from the cliff's crown, she did look, and seeing the distance she'd come—sobriety, finding new friends, ascending this rock—provided its own beautiful, wordless answer.

GLITTERING FERRIS WHEEL

We whiz past the carnival on our way to other (more serious! more responsible!) things; we look in our rearview mirror at a Ferris wheel glittering, Tilt-A-Whirl rides filled with screaming teens, crowds milling through the rusty, spindly, rickety, magical place, eating cotton candy and funnel cakes. (Or in Texas: perfectly fried . . . butter?!)

Dear friends, it's time to take a U-turn.

We are drawn to the music. We wait on line for rides that make our stomachs shiver. We let dusk wash over us, and wander from the Tunnel of Love to a fried Oreo to custom airbrushed T-shirts.

The carnival is such an American dream, sweet as a Kiwi Snow Cone, greasy and delicious like a giant pretzel in the sun, loud and proud, with mechanized melodies playing from every angle, flares and bulbs and beads of light swirling, rides that leave you breathless, games to bet on—and right when you're about to give up, you win the pink teddy bear that barely fits in the trunk of the car.

Carnivals also have that life-in-the-shadows element, the hawkers shouting in an unrelenting voice, the carnival workers staring at you with bloodshot eyes or too much merriment or pure malice. The fair can be an enthrallingly strange place.

Another modern playground is escape rooms. Amanda and her kids tried one: it was a re-creation of the apartment of a 1950s-era spy, complete with mid-century furniture and Russian books. As the clock ticked (the fictional spy would be home in an hour!), they read maps, decoded documents, gasped as walls revealed hidden rooms. Now they seek out escape rooms wherever they go, even bringing boxed "Escape Games" to family gatherings.

We start out life in a sandbox, or on a swing set, and eventually find our way to Meow Wolf's House of Eternal Return in Santa Fe, New Mexico—a twenty-thousand-square-foot complex of dreams, an interactive network of rooms. Being in each chamber is like standing in someone's brain. Jardine was reading a note on the refrigerator in a makeshift kitchen there when suddenly the door opened and a little kid walked out, and she almost fainted. It turns out the fridge is a tunnel to another chamber, and that's the nature of the place. Unexpected worlds lie behind the door of something you think you understand.

At Meow Wolf, she could feel the artist coming up with the idea, because she was inside the idea. She wasn't just looking at it or hearing it. She was immersed in it.

Pop-up installations are spreading like a fever. During the holidays, even the lightscapes made in public parks are a portal to a visionary world. In Marfa, Texas, an art destination at the border of Mexico and Texas, Amanda was gobsmacked by two art installations: Ballroom Marfa's "Hello Meth Lab in the Sun," an installation she walked through (it was built to look like a motel where meth was cooked); and Ilya Kabakov's Russian schoolhouse, which had the air of a place abandoned quickly and fearfully.

Jardine finally made it into the Kusama Infinity Mirror Room when it was installed at the Broad Museum in Los Angeles. It's not a big space, and guests are allowed in a few at a time for only forty seconds. She and her friends waited and waited, and then took their turn. The lights and mirrors, once the door was closed, made an infinity not just of the space but of the day. They multiplied it forever. Even if they had taken a good photograph or video, it could never be true to standing there. In this day and age when everything is documented, to have that ephemeral rapture was a gift, created by a Japanese artist who dreamed it up and made it happen and invited strangers into her imagination.

KARAOKE

Amanda has (very) vague memories of singing karaoke in dim halls and in the corners of bars. Once, she sang "Islands in the Stream" and remembers being awesome, but when she asked a friend to send the video proof, the friend demurred, saying, "Um, you were pretty drunk. I sort of deleted that."

(An aside: As the shame fades, so does the crispness of those old humiliations. This might be one of the best things about sobriety—the ability to process things that happen, and then to "sort of delete it" and move forward, owning it. *Yeah, honey. I sang "Islands in the Stream" and fell off the stage. Everything's copy.*)

A writer Amanda loves and admires came to town during her earliest sober days. As the author signed her newest great book, she leaned close and said, "I'm headed to karaoke with a few friends after this. Join us?"

Amanda stammered. She hemmed and hawed. In her car, clutching the book, she tried to get herself in the mood for sober karaoke.

She started the car. And then, crying, she drove home. It was too much.

This felt like a failure all around, and it just sucked. Amanda ate so many Junior Mints. She did not drink. One day became the next day, and then the next.

A year or so later, another writer she admires came to town. (He is also a close friend, which helped.) Hoping for a redo, Amanda suggested karaoke after his book event and he happily agreed. A few friends joined them in a private karaoke room, ordering champagne and a seltzer water for Amanda.

The pounding of her heart. The taste of Topo Chico with lime. Her famous friend took the microphone, and sang "Pussy Control" by Prince. It was amazing.

Amanda didn't sing right away. She watched and chatted. It was a little bit boring, and a little bit stressful, and she felt the boredom and stress. Finally, full of fear and mozzarella sticks, she stood.

Amanda's sober debut was "Here I Go Again" by Whitesnake. She threw her hair around. She really went for it, especially during the chorus: *Here I GOOOOOOOOOOO!*

To be honest, she rocked that karaoke room. Soon afterward she pulled The Vanish. Driving home, she felt like a fledgling rock star. The famous friend posted a video of Amanda's Whitesnake performance, and it got many likes.

It felt like Amanda was back but also like she was somewhere new entirely. A version of herself she'd always been trying to be, her whole life.

Here we go.

FORMULA 1

ven before Jardine had a clue about the art of the race, the psychopathic nerves-of-steel precision genius of the drivers, the opulent grease-and-gasoline world, she arrived at the track for the first time with her pops and knew immediately that she loved it. It was the inaugural year at Austin's Circuit of the Americas, but while the physical place was new, the rabid fan base was not, and she could smell obsession on the hot Texas wind. Being caught up in the madness and fever of a crowd as maniacal as Formula 1 is a rush, a deliverance to an unexplored plane of existence. Even if it's just for one day.

Her dad is a gearhead and he's always been a lover of F1—he was over the moon when Austin announced a new circuit to the worldwide calendar of grand prix races from Monaco to China to Brazil. So they go together every year. This world of sport comes with a vast web of feuds and alliances between team owners and drivers that is better than any soap opera ever made. It also comes with an international community, so the fans represent all cultures and languages. For chrissake, there are nightclubs that move with the race, being flown from one country to the next. F1 is a universe.

Back in the day, going to the race would have been an all-day and all-night drinking commitment for her, but now Jardine does upon arrival what has become her routine at mega events—she looks at the long long *long* line for overpriced lukewarm beer, then looks at the long long *long* line at the Porta-Potty. Then she thanks herself for jumping off that hamster wheel. But that's it, that's all the time she spends thinking about beer or the lack of it—because she's enveloped and enraptured and engaged, sweating with anxiety and pleasure, watching with everyone, tiers and tiers of spectators all turning as one face, watching Lewis Hamilton blow by, in the lead by a millimeter. His red bumper practically kisses another car as it passes, performing a dangerous takeover like a chess move by a master, and the sponsor emblems gleam and flash on the doors and hoods. A bionic sonic wasp-buzz drones around the track as the cars make another lap, and her dad shouts answers to her questions about the race, while the British sportscaster's voice blooms into the giant sky, and this is just one of those days that needs nothing extra, not a thing, she has it all, and she gets to scream and clap and—of course—root for the underdog.

DONKEY KONG + RED BULL

Come on in! Saunter with us right through the door at Pinballz, a massive building filled to the rafters with games and machines in Austin, busy with friends and strangers on a Saturday night. Enter a zone of electric screens lit up with clown faces and *Raiders of the Lost Ark* and panthers and fairy tales and *Star Wars,* and noises that remind you of a toy shop in outer space, and the smell of old carpet and Skittles and metal and glass and ginger ale. Sit in front of the digital racetrack on a hard-plastic motorcycle, which leans as you ride through a pixelated landscape, the steady hungry thrum of the bike making your heart pound. Spin out, you and the machine crashing and sliding, all kinds of catastrophe and disaster happening in this otherworld, and you get up again. You slurp a milkshake as your rider-surrogate gets going.

When that game is done, you go straight to another game, and then to another. Time feels suspended in arcades, measured out more by quarters than minutes. And everyone here is playing. Look around, darlings. It's playtime all the time. The mechanized claw grabs at magenta bunnies and striped tigers in a glass case. Grown-ups act like kids and kids run wild.

Born an introvert (who loves people, she swears it!), Jardine, even as a four-year-old, was the quiet one in the corner of birthday parties. There's a bit of shame that comes with that territory. To this day, if someone says, "Hey, loosen up," it hits a nerve. "Smile. Don't be so uptight. Why are you so serious?"

Take a guess what helped us out of this little iron collar of self-consciousness—that's right! Booze. *You want me to loosen up? Welllllllll, watch this.* And honestly, we miss that presto-magic–instant option because we did bond with people as we flung ourselves en masse around a dance floor, or giggled uncontrollably together in a ladies' room stall, or staggered down a sidewalk as a pack reliving the highlights and low points of a hilarious night. And being sober now doesn't discredit those times, or those friends, or those dance floors.

But playing Big Buck Hunter as a grown woman, with a Twizzler between her teeth like a cigarillo, cursing and laughing, cheeks flushed with merciless ambition—that's also a proper unloosening. Win or lose, arcades are a *bing-pop-pow* purple-red-orange-lights nasty-sweet anti-uptight time. You can go into an arcade feeling awkward, but you'll always leave undone. You can stay up late and still get up the next beautiful day and feel not just good but great.

IN YOUR GLASS

Drink your tea slowly and reverently,
as if it is the axis on which the world earth revolves—
slowly, evenly, without rushing toward the future.

~THICH NHAT HANH

DECONSTRUCTING
THE HOT TODDY

We still crave liquid comfort—a treat in a glass, a warm drink. Sometimes we want it because we feel under the weather, and sometimes we want it because we feel good. We have a big stoneware mug for this one. We also have a mohair blanket or a terribly behaved and darling puppy or a lover or a very good novel to read. In between loving or reading (or both), we sip our hot toddy.

Jardine used to go to a tiny bar down in TriBeCa, in New York, and the bleached-blonde avant-garde bartender there would make her a hot toddy when she was feeling sick; he'd actually run over to the restaurant next door to grab a pat of butter as the finishing flourish, since this is what his grandmum did in Wales for him as a boy. Jardine will never forget him.

Like many drink recipes, the hot toddy can be broken into basic components so that you can recombine and play with ingredients and create your own mugful. Most hot toddies call for hot liquid, a spray of citrus, a sweetener, and spice (and many include alcohol, but to be frank, they're delicious without it).

How you configure your cup is up to you. For the foundation, you can use hot water, hot tea (Darjeeling, chamomile—whatever you like), or even hot cider. And for citrus, we use Meyer lemon, or blood orange juice, or lime. To sweeten, we can add honey or brown sugar or agave or persimmon syrup. Why not add something special too—grated fresh ginger or star anise, a pinch of red chili flakes or cayenne, turmeric, juniper berries or juniper extract (although not for pregnant women), a lavender sprig, cranberries, a cinnamon stick for stirring—or, as a Welsh grandmum's blessing—a pat of butter.

MIDNIGHT + FIRE

Amanda has never been to Ethiopia, but she's obsessed with the country. She peruses photographs of the art deco buildings of Asmara, dreaming of lingering outside the futurist-style Fiat Tagliero service station at sunset. Closer to home, she's thrilled to be invited to her Ethiopian friend's coffee ceremony. Most Ethiopian restaurants also host coffee ceremonies (called Bunna).

Traditionally, the ceremony begins when a young woman in traditional dress (a white shift with bright embroidery at the sleeves and neckline) washes fresh green coffee beans. Amanda's Ethiopian friend is a guy, however, and performed the ceremony wearing a pressed shirt, slacks, and brand-new sneakers. He placed his ceremonial apparatus on his living room floor, telling the group to imagine the rug was "a bed of scented grasses."

Amanda's friend kept his pan of beans dancing over a blue flame, and they took twenty minutes to roast, filling the air with a dusky, pungent scent that combined with incense burning in the corner of the room. He carried the smoking pan to each of the guests, encouraging everyone to breathe in the smell. He told us he roasted the beans until they were "the perfect color," a deep black-brown, shining with aromatic oils.

Next, he ground the beans with a mortar and long-handed pestle. "This isn't for the weak," he noted.

He added the ground beans and water to his *jebena,* a black clay pot that's round at the bottom and has a straw lid. He placed the *jebena* on the flame, boiling the coffee strong and hot. He loved showing off: he had perfected the art of holding the *jebena* high and pouring a thin stream into each cup.

The first cup is given to the eldest in the room. It tasted of midnight and fire.

IMPERIAL DRAGONWELL

On a road trip through Santa Fe, Jardine stopped at a tea shop, and just standing in that room—with hundreds of tea canisters, hand-lettered with names, on all the shelves—was a daylight seduction. The words alone—Blackwood Ceylon, Heavenly Blue Peak, Himalayan Snowflake, Volcano Flower Burst—made a sort of poetic and culinary pornography. She grinned in earnest delight.

With tea, there is ceremony, and there is nuance. There is inhaling the divine steam rolling up from the cup. There is sharing, there is giving. There can be daydreaming and there can be letting go.

We love the glass teapots that show a jasmine bud, dried hard and tight into a ball, blossom slowly in the hot water. It looks like a wild and dangerous heart.

We love the lexicon of ingredients, from the Sicilian blood orange infusion, to the honeysuckle note in the white tea called Silver Needle from China, to the Ti Kuan Yon tea that has a trace of orchid perfume in it, to the Baroness Grey, which is Earl Grey with piquant lemon. Amanda discovered the smoky appeal of artichoke tea at a writing retreat and now orders it from London.

We buy cheap nameless tea in a paper cup when we're in a rush. We sometimes make tea at home for a friend, with an almond biscuit, and serve it in a cup (inherited from a grandmother) whose ceramic is so thin that sunlight shines through the rim. On days when we're writing up a storm and crave something—anything—we go through a pot or two of lemongrass tea. When we're afraid we might not sleep, we fall back on the old nighttime teas that feel like a mother kissing your forehead. Amanda loves caramel chamomile and lavender with rooibos. (They sound fancy, but they're both supermarket mixes that come in boxes featuring a bear wearing a sleeping cap.)

As with so many things, too, sometimes it's enough to stand in a tea shop, see the shelves and shelves of loveliness, and walk out empty-handed and awakened.

DECONSTRUCTING
THE BLOODY MARY

There's nothing like a Bloody Mary—it sits in its own category, gloriously alone, coral-red and flecked with horseradish, crowned with salt, speared with a celery stalk, and spritzed with lime. But that's just the template—there's an infinity of permutations on the classic tomato-juice cocktail. They're often just as good without booze *and* they're a perfect drink if you're hungry.

There's a bunch of formal iterations: like the Bloody Caesar (with Clamato), or the Bloody Maria (with a Mexican slant, like jalapeños). Or you can get to know the building blocks for Bloody Mary ingredients and construct your own.

Riffs on the drink can start with tomato juice, adding or substituting one of these: olive brine, clam broth, lemon juice, Worcestershire, green tomatillo juice, squid ink, beet juice, sriracha, pickle juice, pho broth, white balsamic, miso, tomato water, fish sauce, or one of any number of Bloody Mary mixes you can snag off the grocery-store shelf.

And then there's the spice and herb factor—you can play by mixing in or rimming the glass with black pepper, cilantro, paprika, basil, cayenne, fennel seeds, grapefruit zest, wasabi, Himalayan salt, truffle powder, minced ginger, sesame oil, dill, or celery salt.

And *then,* dear friends, there's the GARNISH. We're open to endless variations starting with okra, bacon, artichoke hearts, smoked oysters, pickled carrots, Greek olives, kimchi, crawfish, wild scallion, beef jerky, a blood orange wedge, mozzarella balls, a sprig of rosemary, or yellow pepper. We've even seen a cheeseburger speared on a wooden stake atop a Bloody Mary's pint glass.

You can find a bursting library of recipes online for Bloody Marys, from the simplest and most classic, to out-there and psychedelic ideas, to little elegant smart twists that are seasonal or in honor of an iconic soul. And the Bloody Mary is visually impactful. This drink is a still-life painting in its statuesque presentation of tomato and fish and leaf, or a Dali-esque conglomeration of symbols, of radishes and shrimp melting over the rim of the glass with a surreal slyness. This zero-proof cocktail welcomes all food groups and can channel the spirit of any culture or country. You can experiment with rare and poetic possibilities, or just check what's in the fridge today.

Our vodka-full Bloody Marys of yesterday, though, were always good for marking memories, thumbtacking them to the bulletin board in our minds. This made us reluctant to let go of them, as if the memory (of our parents playing afternoon backgammon when we were little, of New Year's Day brunch with a new boyfriend in Brooklyn, of a boat ride to Fire Island with friends) would vanish without the Bloody Mary to pin it down.

We're not wrong in that so many intense moments of our lives have been secured by what we were drinking or eating—what we shared with friends and family—what loved ones served us. Like mint tea in Marrakech, or the powdery spicy Russian tea cookie our grandmother made, or the fried avocado we ate with our best girlfriends when we were eighteen and road-tripping through California, or the V8 on the rocks we always have on airplanes because it signals new ideas, possibilities, horizons.

Food and drink do mark experiences and memories, they do embody the love between people, the excitement of traveling, the generosity of hospitality, exchanges that have been happening since the dawn of humankind and will always be precious and important. They are cues to places, people, moments. But nowhere does it say they must be alcoholic.

SPRINGTIME GREEN JUICE

Jardine doesn't have the most impeccable track record when it comes to hydration. Back in high school, she'd stumble out of lacrosse practice, and her replenishment of choice was a Welch's grape soda, chilled and dewy from the vending machine. *Water, what's that?* She went to a doctor in her midtwenties complaining of a never-ending headache, and for her to go to a doctor at all, to notice something amiss AT ALL, in those days, when she was absolutely disconnected from her physical well-being, was amazing, so it was a real headache. The doctor asked if she was drinking enough water. *Why would I drink water,* she asked, *when I have coffee, Mountain Dew, and Johnny Walker Red?* She looks back and sees she lived at least one solid decade permanently dehydrated.

So it makes sense that she used to LOVE to make fun of people who got wheatgrass shots and who blitzed concoctions in special blenders, because they were being so precious. Getting sober, though, has involved poking and prodding the arguments we made over the years. We used to believe that taking care of our health was narcissistic—but somehow getting wasted and then being useless the next day was compassionately going to save the world? What's more self-involved than a hangover? Bad hangovers did sometimes allow for commiseration and connection among friends and coworkers, but it's strange logic to think it was "selfless" to be damaged.

Some juice shops are highway robbery, just sugar water and a manipulation of ideas about self-worth on the label. But we've fallen in love with the good joints that serve brilliant poems of drinks, lyrical potions, magic spells of spices and fruit and oils and vegetables.

We honestly don't know our turmeric from our spirulina, so this is not a recommendation of anything in particular. But hopefully you'll get the same sensation we do, of light and energy in our cells, like the power of photosynthesis.

FLOWERS IN YOUR CUP

Summertime is here, and there's a disco party in the garden tonight! Fireflies, gold pollen, and perfume, a blossom here and leaf there, a secret Eden in our glass . . .

We love to mix herbs and flowers and fruits into our drinks. For distilling the garden into your cup, there are sacred texts from centuries past about which root or seed to use, for hedonistic or medicinal purposes, and an ever-expanding world of techniques and ideas offered online. (Guidance from expert consultants is essential, too, since we can't just forage for anything pretty in the backyard or we'll have *Blue Lagoon* on our hands!)

We can make tisanes or infusions from lemongrass or wild rose petals or raspberries, steeping the ingredient in hot water and then straining the liquid for a basic botanical element to any drink. Freeze edible flowers in ice cubes, or suspend them in pastel Jell-O squares. We can float a transparently thin slice of preserved apple or dried pear on top of a drink. Muddle strawberries or dill in a pint glass and add seltzer or ginger brew or cold tea. We can make floral simple syrups, steeping elderflower or lavender in sugar and water and then straining that too.

We can perch a tiny French violet candy or sugar-crystallized Sweet William at the top of a rocks glass.

We can pair rosewater and mint, or make a trinity of sage and lemon and honey.

Use lilac blossoms for ice cream, then create a ginger-beer float with a pale purple scoop.

Pile fresh fruit into your drinks, kiwi slices and pieces of cantaloupe, and wild blueberries picked that morning. We can make flower Popsicles to dip into our passion-fruit lassi. We can throw rose petals on top of a zero-proof cocktail, or scatter flowers over a punch bowl, or toss them in a silver ice bucket.

An orchid in a goblet is especially cinematic—once you've sipped your drink, you can tuck the sticky, wild, tropical, redolent blossom behind your ear.

DECONSTRUCTING FALL DRINKS

What do we want in an autumn drink? The sparkle of a dark rain, mysteries stored in dank, shadowy piles of leaves, a pale sun, tweed coats, orchards, being chilly on a screened-in porch, collecting firewood, polishing leather boots that have been in the attic all summer, coziness, sap, cashmere, spice, comfort, love.

Here's a little cabinet of ingredients: apple cider, ginger, cranberry, peppermint, fennel, pomegranate, saffron, maple, quince, chai tea, thyme, cinnamon, pear, anise, pumpkin spice, cardamom, fig, rosemary, cloves, orange wedge, turmeric, ginger beer, Earl Grey tea.

Cinnamon variations alone are worth exploring, since this barklike spice can taste different depending on if it came from Indonesia or Sri Lanka or China or Saigon. Ginger beers have proliferated in the last decade, so there's a spectrum of heat and tang to them, and they're always an easy base to have on hand. Cider is a good base, too, hot or cold. The beauty of heating it is in making the home smell like heaven. Fall drinks can be complex and botanical, with homemade thyme syrup and a dollop of persimmon paste stirred into seltzer and garnished with pickled blood orange, or they can be simple: cardamom tea steeped then chilled over ice.

Fall is a time of transition, as every season is in its way, but here we see things falling, burning out, becoming ash, going to sleep. These drinks are a way to savor the taste and memories of this season, to hold that moment in time on our tongue, to be part of the metamorphosis.

TINY ODE TO WATER

Mineral water, tap water, sparkling water, glacier water, purified water, cold water, ice water, alkaline water, spring water, distilled water, water infused with cucumber or mint or lemon or pineapple or basil or ginger or thyme or kiwi or strawberry, Pellegrino, Perrier, Voss Sparkling Water, water in a crystal glass, water from a garden hose, water in a Dixie cup, water scooped up in your hands, water after running, after walking in the sun, after skiing, after a sauna, after waking up, water in the middle of the night, water after sweating, after crying, after sex, water on the airplane, water in the car, water coolers at work, water fountains at parks, Topo Chico, Adirondack Seltzer, Waterloo Sparkling Watermelon, Vittel, Mountain Valley Spring Water, Evian, Dasani, water on your lips, water down your throat, water through your whole beautiful body to flush it out and protect your spinal cord and help you think and stay cool or warm and be well, BPA-free plastic or no-break glass or stainless steel bottles to carry everywhere so (mwah ha ha!) you shall not have to pay the ridiculous prices of water bottles and create more plastic in the world and you can put stickers all over them like you're still in tenth grade, water from the sky, from the ground, getting drenched, getting quenched—dear dear H2O, you are part of us, moving through our bloodstreams and cells, you make up more than 60 percent of our bodies at any given time, and we adore you.

DECONSTRUCTING EGGNOG

Supermarket eggnog is gnarly, but Jardine looooov-vvvvveeeessss it. Or she loves two or three sips of it every December, and then she has to lie down in a fetal state and live out her stomachache. It's some weird stuff. A goopy drink that's sort of the pale thick creamy yellow of a Texas sky in winter.

But that's talking about store-bought, and this is one of those drinks that can take many forms if you do it at home. It can be the airy fluffy creamy stuff of angels, or a vegan ambrosia with coconut milk and Medjool dates and ground cloves. It falls into that milk and honey world, stirring up the idea of delight. The basic procedure involves milk, eggs, sugar. And then you can crush crystallized ginger on top, or swirl in melted dark chocolate, drizzle in maple syrup, stir it with a cinnamon stick or candy cane, place a spear of preserved cherries or plump dried apricots on the top, or dust it with nutmeg. Jardine is pretty pagan, so for her the drink is not about a specific holiday as much as it's about snow and mittens and darkness falling very early and a cold landscape gleaming out of a window. It's a potion for innocence. To be poured after sledding.

If you're hosting a party and serving eggnog, and you decide to make one batch with alcohol and the other without—this can be lovely and also tricky. For sober people, a little mistake like sipping an alcoholic eggnog could be devastating. So making place cards that say what's what is essential. (And as an imbiber at a big party, being careful about where we put our glass down and which glass we pick up is also a thing.)

This differentiation is a priority when hosting any event where mixed drinks are presented in punch bowls or carafes, and some include booze and some do not. It's getting more and more acceptable—wait, it's more than acceptable, it's now actually, believe it or not, *cool!*—to name a drink with a placard and to be forthright about its alcohol content and lack thereof. (It used to be that if you were sober and you showed up at a party, someone related to the host would hustle you into a back room and slip you a club soda disguised as a gin and tonic in such a shady, shameful way that you knew it was an embarrassment to all involved, mostly yourself.) Now, with beautiful culinary magazines running pieces on botanical zero-proof drinks, and avant-garde influencers blazing new trails in entertainment and hosting, and clubs with zero-proof nights that are superchic, it's possible to put the nonalcoholic drinks at the front. To show them off.

LOVE

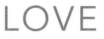

Love makes your soul crawl out from its hiding place.

~ZORA NEALE HURSTON

BINGSU + MINIATURE GOLF: THE ART OF THE SOBER DATE

Our earliest memories about flirting take place in the middle-school gym, at the neighborhood swimming pool, hanging outside the 7-Eleven and watching skateboarders and trying to look bored, and they feature blushing till our ears were scarlet, avoiding whoever we were crushing on, furtively scribbling in diaries, whispering with friends, dying inside, and simultaneously feeling intolerably alive.

Not much changed as Jardine got older and theoretically wiser. Dating still felt dangerous, vulnerable, and thrilling, but more than anything, like a game that other people knew how to play and she didn't. One solution was to drink and get high while dating, and her relationships often revolved around drinking because that's where the relationship started and how the relationship came to be. Funny that the thing we search for, that hammering heart, that rush of blood and heat through the system, is sometimes exactly what we'd dilute by getting drunk. Isn't all that bananas-crazy energy what we live for?

One of the most formidable stumbling blocks when we first considered sobriety was fearing that without booze, we didn't know how to find someone to date and love, or how to hang out, or how to hook up. We thought courtship minus substances wasn't possible.

How do we get from the first hello to the thumping heart, from swipe-right to meeting at a restaurant, from the pause in conversation to the first kiss, not to mention *even consider* getting naked? It's hard to step out into the world when we quite obviously want something and yet we're unprotected by a veil of intoxication.

Some people love the first date, and it's date number six or seven when things get real and complex and uncomfortable for them. But for many of us, the first date is brutal. It's an experiment in radical vulnerability. Instead of seeing such an experiment as negative, we're trying to dip into it these days, be exhilarated by it.

We used to drink wine while getting ready, then meet our date at a bar, drink through dinner, then go to another bar, *finis*. We'd wake up in someone's bed, or on our couch, clothes still damp from making out in the rain—a phone number written on our palm but other details missing. Over Advil and mimosas, we'd plan with our best friend what came next.

Chemicals were a way to fast-forward through the awkward stages of dating someone new. It seemed otherwise impossible to move from being alone, staring at a text or a digital profile, toward that place of abandon where we wanted to be. Or, worse, to tolerate coming home alone AGAIN when the date was a bomb. This is rough and raw stuff.

Jardine was single when she got sober, and she shyly reluctantly nervously *finally* made an online dating profile. She checked the box for *sober* herself, and wrote that it was a priority, and she also clicked it as a priority in whoever she was seeking. A sober guy who lived in Austin, too, and taught wood shop and was wearing pine-green corduroys in his photo started corresponding with her, so they met for coffee. They made clumsy conversation. He was starving, and she wasn't, so she watched him wolf down a big plate of eggs.

He apologized for being so hungry, and she laughed because he was funny, and they decided to make another date.

He'd had more time sober, and more practice at sober dating, so when he came to get her in his banged-up silver truck, he already knew where they were going. Dinner at a vegetarian Italian joint, then on to pinball and Red Bulls, then an old-school soda fountain for ice cream. They hung out for hours, and he kissed her when he dropped her off. It was superfun, and yet Jardine balked at how close they'd felt, the "ordinary intimacy" that was so different from the one-night stand, and almost more painful to handle. She hid, and they didn't keep dating, but she felt empowered from the experience. They decided to be friends, and hung out for a year before they fell in love, and started a relationship that thrives to this day.

Maybe those uncomfortable places that occur in early dating are building blocks to a strong bond. Maybe good things take time. Maybe we *have* to go out into the world before we know what we want if we're going to get what we want.

Amanda was long married with three kids when she got sober. "Date night" always meant escape and reconnection, a time to remember who she and her husband were as lovers and adults, a time to find "fun." Opportunities were limited: sitters are expensive and life is overfull. A few quick drinks made Amanda shed her mom-self and connect to her sweet husband. They stayed close to home, lingering at expensive restaurants with cheap happy hours.

When Amanda stopped drinking, everything had to change. Amanda could no longer switch between selves so easily. She felt awkward too—confused, sad, yearning. She needed to plan better—to seek out art museums and comedy shows, to change "date night" to "Sunday morning, no-kid hike with time to talk and lie in the sunshine." To spend the money she once blew on cocktails on a hotel room with a view that she and her husband would only use for a few fabulous hours.

If we could tell our past selves some things about dating sober, the first thing we would say is: You will be vulnerable, you will get yourself into real situations where there's nowhere to hide. But that might be the best thing that ever happened.

We'd say: Don't be afraid of the gentleman or lady who seems to be a full-on dork when they suggest ideas for your date like miniature golf and Bingsu (Korean shaved ice), or a Oaxacan dinner and laser tag, or just wandering a neighborhood neither of you know and seeing what turns up. Or on the other hand, if he or she balks at your proposal of a late-night swim and lying in the grass and looking at stars instead of pounding shots at a bar, that ain't a good sign for the future.

We'd say: tell this new person early on that you don't drink and put the sober thing out there instead of lugging it around like a rock secretly strapped to your back.

We'd tell her: You're going to feel intense waves of emotion during a date. Instead of breaking down and ordering a drink, head to the bathroom and splash water on your face. Call a sober friend or just breathe slowly. You're allowed to simply go home. You can text your people and laugh about it, hash it out, or write it up in your notebook as a ridiculous story. We'd remind her that falling into bed by ourselves after a failed date was not as lonely as waking up with someone we really didn't dig, hungover to death. Being drunk and estranged from your own heart is the pinnacle of being alone. Please don't do that anymore.

Last we'd say: Baby girl, you know you're allowed to fall in love, right?

SEX SHOP

We've driven past it a hundred times. Maybe we've popped in—but just to the front of the store, we're sure no one saw us—to buy penis straws for a bachelorette party, or edible underwear, or elephant pants with a very special trunk. We've giggled as we paused by the glass windows. But now it's time to go inside. Deep inside.

Amanda parked at Bird's Barber Shop and then, eyes darting both ways, walk-jogged past Aviary wine bar (her old haunt) and Black Sheep Lodge (oh, she'd had a late-night beer or four there). Why she'd never felt shame overdrinking in these local hot spots but felt such trepidation entering Cindie's (Number One in Fantasy and Fun!) was an issue to explore at another time. Because the red-neon Cindie's sign was beckoning.

Amanda pushed open the door.

"Hey there!" called a young woman behind the counter. "You need anything specific?"

A childhood in Catholic Sunday School made Amanda freeze. She just shook her head mutely.

"Well, you let me know!" said the salesclerk.

How Amanda envied her breezy self-confidence! Murmuring, *Oh my,* and *Oh dear,* and *Oh my!* in her mind (but not uttering a sound), Amanda picked up vibrators and cock rings and strap-ons. The voice of her Confraternity of Christian Doctrine teacher at Sacred Heart intoned with disgust: *Amanda, this is not for you.*

But what if it was? What if it could be?

Maybe we *do* want to take a pole-dancing class or surprise our lover with tickets to a burlesque show. Schedule boudoir photo shoots in latex and lace. There are thousands of videos online to check out, to feel good, to find out what we like. One bookworm friend has sworn off literary novels, cuddling at night with juicy erotic ones—anything by Christina Lauren. ("They're positively loin-burning!" she confides.)

At Cindie's, Amanda moved on to lingerie. She normally favored silk men's pajamas and Gap Body supersoft nightgowns. She'd tried to wear a thong in the early 2000s but never got used to it the way her sexier friends promised. Amanda's thoughts on panty lines were, *Why ya lookin'?*

Could Amanda put on these thigh-high patent leather snow-white stiletto boots and try out the whip in the mirror? She swallowed. A gaggle of confident millennials entered the store. When the clerk cried, "Hey, girls!" they went straight to the counter and told her what they wanted—chins up, eyes clear. The clerk packaged their toys in brown paper bags (like the ones Amanda had used for her children's lunches before she got into sober self-care and told them to pack their own lunches). Amanda coveted the young women's easy sexuality, their straight bangs, the high-waisted "mom jeans" that—against all odds—looked awesome.

Amanda gathered a satin negligee and stilettos, lifting her own chin and smiling as she passed the youngsters on the way to the dressing room.

"Have fun in there!" said the salesclerk.

Amanda swallowed but did not stop.

And let's just say she left Cindie's with her own brown paper bag.

THE ANSWER IS YES

David Foster Wallace, a writer we love and mourn, once told a joke to a reporter:

"What does a writer say after sex?"

"Was it as good for me as it was for you?"

Many of us have forgotten to ask if things are good for us. We don't even know what we enjoy or want—we're disconnected from ourselves. Sometimes, drinking allowed us to stay in the wrong lives. It's scary as f*%k to blow up your life. For some of us, getting sober meant valuing ourselves more than others for the very first time.

This is a terrifying thing to do—we used to find it way more socially acceptable to please everyone else, to be liked, to avoid rocking the boat at all costs. Sometimes we drank to make others feel OK. Sometimes we drank to mask the fact that we were not OK, that one thing (or everything) needed to change.

It felt subversive to finally ask, What *is* good for us? Who do *we* want to be? What do we like? Who makes us feel valued and safe? How do we make the hours beautiful, the days and nights beautiful, the weeks and months and years of our life beautiful? What feels nice? What makes us purr? If we break it down, molecule by molecule, where does our pleasure begin? Did we really have fun? Was it as good for us as it was for you? Did I wake up bedraggled or radiant? What does that say about what happened? Are we ready to deal with that question honestly?

Is our most shining, most beautiful self sober? Is this good for me?

For us, the answer is yes.

DIGITAL ORCHIDS

n sobriety we sometimes get tunnel vision and look too hard for the giant solution to connection, the big and absolute fix to loneliness, when it might pay to send out tiny gossamer threads of affection instead.

Jardine's friend Johnny, who lives across the country, texts her a word-of-the-day out of the blue. A few recent examples: *fulgurant* (adjective): flashing like lightning; *dégringolade* (noun): a rapid decline or deterioration (as in strength, position, or condition); *addlepated* (adjective): 1. being mixed up, confused; 2. eccentric.

She loves this. She loves getting a mini-missive from a friend. An uncomplicated note that keeps them in touch.

It feels as good to send as to receive, so she likes to reach out to everyone, anyone. Send something spontaneous, silly, dear, and only if it's a pleasure and not a chore. E-mail a friend a photo-booth strip you took together back in the day. Send a Warsan Shire poem to someone. A Magnum PI gif to your mother who doesn't know what a gif is but sure does like her some Tom Selleck. Just send out a text message to friends you miss on a regular old Wednesday morning.

If done with presence of mind, and not just thrown like a desperate net to catch attention, or an emotional booty call to ten targets (*um, how does Jardine know that this version happens? because she's done it*), it can be a sweet way to connect, or pay forward some love.

So many times, she's gotten a photo from a friend that made her smile and stop and pay attention. It feels different from seeing things on social media. Jardine's friend Beth sends her photos of almost-dead orchids she finds on the street in San Francisco, plants that people have given up on, which then Beth takes home and brings back to life. Her friend Bruce sends her surreal collages of cats in Brooklyn apartments. Her friend Melissa sends links to books she might adore. Nothing that requires a text or e-mail back. Just little kisses blown through the air.

Jardine had a revelation one year in college—it was Valentine's Day and she was wistfully waiting for a gift or card or invite or something from anyone, and she suddenly saw how passive she was being. Why not be the one to send the card, make the call, leave a rose on someone's doorstep, or at the very least, text a Mapplethorpe photo of a calla lily to someone, which is like leaving it on his or her digital doorstep? There's a meditation where you go through people in your life and spend a moment wishing each one happiness. Amazing how these things—putting love out there instead of waiting for it—can jack up a bad mood better than anything.

CRUSH

One of our greatest revelations about being sober was that *sober* doesn't mean "straitlaced." It doesn't mean "obedient." *Sober* doesn't mean "prim." It actually allows us more bandwidth for risk. Dear heavens, if we could send a postcard to our twenty-five-year-old self, who was confused and hungover and unhappy, or sober and bored as hell, it would have this message scrawled on it with twenty exclamation marks: sobriety can make room for *more* wildness, more fantasy, more crushes.

As with so much stuff on the sober side of life, it's easy to turn an innocent (and innocently dirty) thing into an addiction, and we've seen people switch up a reliance on liquor to a dependence on sex—using it to feel high, to feel anything, to make a connection with anyone. If we notice we're doing something compulsively, we step back. But there's a good distance between playfully stirring the imagination and libido—and being destructively pathological.

What was your first crush? Do you remember it? Jardine has little avalanches of images, sun streaming through a smeared winter school-bus window, her heart beating double-time, her crush sitting one seat away, the world outside moving slow as honey while the cozy interior of that bus became everything and everywhere; nothing else mattered.

Why not allow that energy to run through our circuitry these days? Can we access that raw and gorgeous thrill? If we're single, let it burn and then turn into something more, or not. If we're in a relationship, the outside crush can fuel the commitment. If we're polyamorous, it can spin the globe in our hands.

We can have crushes on officemates and next-door neighbors, or movie stars, or people who don't even exist, like characters from books. We can have crushes on men or women, they can be sexual or platonic crushes, we don't need to be in control of them, and when they die out, we can be sad for a few days. They're small fires in the soul, shooting stars, not meant to last, breathtaking because of their brevity.

When we were party monsters and heavy drinkers and often hungover, we had a compromised distribution system for energy. Some of it surely went to crushes, but a lot went to shame and protecting the self that had been dangerously exposed, to putting back the pieces after benders. Now we have a little extra fuel to burn because there isn't this leak in the pipe. To be honest, this surplus was one of the most unexpected parts of the sober experiment.

LIKE A VIRGIN

et's just say that much of our sensual lives was dipped in booze, even waterlogged in it, over the years. But getting sober, and then getting naked sober, and realizing it would be a lucid experience from here on, no blurry vision or spotty memory to hide behind—that brought on a moment of reckoning. We thought, *Wow, you have to be seriously bold to have sex sober*, and then we thought, *But why exactly, when you've been having sex for years, and it's not like you don't know what happens next? What specifically are you afraid of?* Good question.

It's easy for a sober sexual experience to feel like the very first time, we've found, over and over. All the mean girls in our heads keep clanging, a bell of eighth-grade-cafeteria misery, as we evaluate ourselves in the medicine-cabinet mirror while someone waits in the bedroom. Maybe we look at our bodies and tighten the belt on our robe instead of untying it. Maybe we dab on a bit of rose lipstick and some musky perfume, trying to see a renegade sex-machine in our reflection. We might try to remember X-rated tips we read somewhere, or drum up a few nasty brilliant one-liners worthy of an erotica superstar. Maybe we text a friend to say we're thinking about becoming celibate.

The only way out, our friend might text back, *is to strip down and go back into the bedroom.*

That's not how the saying goes, we write.

Stop texting, the friend writes back.

We might then inhale. Click the light off in the bathroom and float, uncertain and self-conscious, tender and fragile, into the bedroom. The moon might be big out the window. Our heart hammers in our ears, and we suddenly remember everything we'd forgotten, and we say what we really mean:

"Kiss me."

TINY MAGIC
CONNECTIONS

Some people go to priests;
others to poetry;
I to my friends.

~VIRGINIA WOOLF

BEAUTIFUL BEASTS

JIGSAW

REVENGE OF THE NERDS

ERRANDS

TRADER JOE'S COOKIES + A RED TRICYCLE

NIGHT-BLOOMING CEREUS + WOLF MOONS

BROOKLYN BARBERS + STRANGERS IN SCOTLAND

SAGE, EGG SANDWICHES + LOCAL PLUMS

SUPPER CLUBS + STAINED GLASS

BEAUTIFUL BEASTS

What on earth would we do without them? The angel-fish and dogs and cats and snakes and white rats and horses and guinea pigs and rabbits and turtles that share our homes and our lives and our hearts and our souls? "Dogs possess a quality that's rare among humans—the ability to make you feel valued just by being you—and it was something of a miracle to me to be on the receiving end of all that acceptance," writes Caroline Knapp in her memoir *Pack of Two: The Intricate Bond Between People and Dogs.*

Jardine remembers a Wyoming morning when she mounted a horse for the first time in many years and felt tears in her throat, then she was bawling. It came on fast and did not make sense. She had a visceral sense of the horse's kindness: he took her up and down narrow, rocky mountain paths even though Jardine surely transmitted fear and total incompetence through her body, and the horse could have reacted. The horse's calm didn't seem to come from being docile but from being generous. Luckily Jardine was wearing big black sunglasses, and the tears dried up anyway, since she was in this red-rock, blue-sky paradise with a beautiful beast and it was impossible not to grin like a fool.

For seventeen years, Jardine had a ragged anarchist rock star of a toy poodle named Zoe (who came into her life when Jardine was twenty-three and Zoe was eight weeks old) and Jardine loved that little one beyond words. Zoe had a front-row seat to Jardine's messy not-sober life, and never left Jardine's side, and never loved her any less, no matter what condition Jardine was in when she came home.

Jardine's partner, Neil, had a sleek, elegant mutt, Olive, who saw him through addiction, and then also saw him recover. When Neil relapsed once, she panicked and wouldn't come into the house. Animals feel everything. "To endow animals with human emotions has long been a scientific taboo," writes Frans de Waal. "But if we do not, we risk missing something fundamental, about both animals and us."

Even if you can't commit full-time, shelters desperately need people to foster dogs and cats. Many of our friends love to do this. You can also volunteer at stables or pounds or rescue operations, walk a pup on your lunch break, or hang out with one for a few hours on the weekend. To get that animalistic connection happening. Sometimes, animals are wiser and kinder than anyone we know, including ourselves, and they don't care what channel we're watching or what bag of chips we're devouring or what chore we're ignoring as long as we want to cuddle with them.

Amanda is still surprised, every morning, to find herself in thrall to a tiny black schnauzer named Schneffles (after Mount Sneffles in Colorado). But from the moment Neffie rushes to give Amanda her wake-up kiss, with her impossibly fluffy sweet face, through the afternoon—Amanda typing and Neffie snoozing at her side—to the evening, when a walk with Neffie saves Amanda from happy-hour cravings, it's love. And then, lights out, Neff places her paw on Amanda's arm: *I'm here. You can sleep.*

JIGSAW

When Amanda got sober, she knew she didn't want to be stuck at the dinner table or in the living room when her friends and family members were a few drinks in. Her true heart told her to *get out*. But where the heck was she supposed to go?

One winter vacation, Amanda looked up from the grown-ups' table and saw that her children were already in pajamas and gathered around a jigsaw puzzle across the room, laughing and sipping apple cider. She stood, and as if in a trance, walked toward the kids. Their puzzle featured a medley of 1980s candy wrappers. Amanda saw a yellow piece that would fit perfectly in a Sugar Daddy wrapper. "Can I join you?" she asked, and the wonderful children said yes.

Now she often keeps a jigsaw puzzle going during parties. If she feels strange, she can sit and move pieces around. It's a way to be somewhat alone but still in the room.

Hanging out with children—not just watching over them but being on their level—is a fantastic way to change the course of a day.

Amanda takes the kids to the beach while the other adults sleep in, or goes sledding with them after lunch, or strolls the neighborhood with her daughter right around happy hour. And there's nothing more magical than asking a crew of kids, "Anyone want to go for a late-night swim under the stars?"

Even as she sits here typing, Amanda can remember the cheers.

Some of us stopped having fun too early (or never had childhoods where fun was available), or just forgot along the way what it felt like to be un-self-conscious and completely immersed in a game or puzzle or fort or trampoline. And the hyper-creative, sober people who can best teach us how to do it all again are often kids. Amanda's got amazing kids of her very own, and Jardine gets to hang with her awesome nieces and nephew, and her friends' sweet kids. They're wise souls who demonstrate the best way to climb a waterslide, how to tell ghost stories, and how to make s'mores and get the s'mores all over our faces and then make more s'mores. They remind us to sing off-key and really loud, as long as it's from the heart. They can show us how to paint with our fingers, *and* help us see that this blur of black and yellow paint is actually a tiger.

REVENGE OF THE NERDS

We were nerds as kids, and knew we were nerds, and yet we sort of buried our nerdy side as we grew up. We got sober, and it's true, we hunkered down and read murder mysteries and ate supermarket cupcakes and watched *Eastbound & Down* for hours. We might have stayed in the "cozy zone" for weeks, months, even years. And that's fine. But then we peeked up from our nests, hungry for something else.

A new appetite was brewing, but in a way it was just a return to a seminal curiosity, the resurrection of a dorky fixation on a variety of subjects. Amanda took a class on color theory and then joined all the art museums in Austin. She met Jardine for a double date at the Jones Center on a special Members Night where they toured the new exhibits, then stood with their men and gazed at the sun setting over Congress Avenue, and then talked about the show over pasta and bubbly water at an Italian restaurant down the block. (A double date called for four desserts, as well.) At a lecture about how Ellsworth Kelly was inspired by birds, Amanda sat in the front row. She heard a talk on landscape design, and one about making *mole*. (That class taught her she's probably never going to make *mole*.)

Both sober and drinking friends dig museum nights, art talks, film talks, science talks, readings, cooking classes, writing workshops, photography lessons—these are buzzy interactive incubation-spaces for friendships once nurtured in a bar.

We've developed a supersonic sense of things happening near us, whereas we used to be somewhat deaf to it. We've learned to get a yearly membership to places like botanical gardens and space museums for the same price of a single long night's bar tab. We scan the paper and subscribe to local e-mail-newsletters, circling flamenco classes or clicking on collector talks on Betty Sayre or Shirin Neshat. We go to serious lectures and ridiculous lectures and useful talks and esoteric talks, and we know we're in the right room when the person sharing their knowledge is bonkers-in-love with the subject, giddy and generous to be discussing it. We'll listen to almost anything—almost—if the speaker is earnest, because good nerd energy can help us combat a cynical world.

Jardine went to a class taught by a mother and daughter who had followed their (now deceased) leader on pilgrimages for decades; they sat Jardine and her cousin at a small desk, gave them grape juice and cookies, and explained their new religion on a chalkboard. The women looked alike, hair braided down their backs, their tunics part nun's clothes and part 1960s-California-hippie. The afternoon was an education in many things. Jardine and her cousin walked out into a world of rosebushes and smog and chain-link fences and pit bulls and cars, speechless, their minds swimming with biblical diagrams and seeds from bushes in Jerusalem and ivory rosaries and the ideology of these pilgrims. They talked about what they learned, and decided the lesson was that we all believe in something, don't we?

ERRANDS

When Jardine was little, she'd go with her mom to do errands, almost all of which were on the main street of her small town. The dry cleaner, the butcher, the stationery store, the farm stand, the pharmacy, the fishmonger, the bookshop (this was an essential place for her mom, not a luxury), and the hardware shop.

And it's not just that her mom supported her town, or wanted to get out of the house. Her mother actually learned about marinade from the German butcher who wrapped the family's steaks in white paper for years. The fisherman on the wharf not only told her a bayman's tips for grilling bluefish, he would prepare her favorite chowder in bulk for a party, and call her when fresh littleneck clams came in on a boat. The pharmacist would talk to her mother at length; she was generous with her time, making sure she explained everything about a medicine.

Nowadays there's Amazon Prime, the big shopkeep in the sky, and Instacart, and all the permutations of "shopping without leaving your desk." Which, honestly, is a godsend when there's a deadline and a child home sick from school. (Or even when nothing much is keeping you from going out into the world that day except a desire to not go out into the world that day.) And how excellent it can feel to use these new services that have bloomed into our reality.

But it's also grounding and warm to go out and deal with human beings, ask advice, connect over the weather or gossip, as humans have been doing for thousands of years. Man, it can feel lonely to work at home, cut off from anyone except people contacted through technology, or to commute and come home to your apartment without knowing a soul within a three-mile radius. Especially if you no longer hit up the dive bar down the street.

The idea of getting to know local proprietors is almost too obvious, and Jardine is quick to overlook it. But then some Saturday, she ventures out to buy ceramic pots for her new plants. She ends up in a tiny shop around the corner that she never really noticed, and starts talking to the woman who owns it, and hears about her plants and Jardine tells her about her own plants and the woman tells Jardine tricks to growing mint in this climate, then somehow they're talking about California art school in the '80s and Eve Babitz and the best Thai place nearby and what to order (a dish with preserved kaffir limes that isn't on the menu, but she's friends with the chef and he loves to cook it), and Jardine walks out, dazed with friendliness, with two turquoise pots that have the right drainage for her plants, three new ideas about what to do in her hood, and a little more pop in her step.

Granted, we've also gone the brick-and-mortar route only to deal with a total asshole. But there's something about the ornery old dude at the shoe repair place—beware, sometimes he's a new friend in disguise, testing you with his misanthropic skit to see who you are. If you make it past the barrier, you might suddenly have a link to the legends and secrets of your town, to wisdom about life (and penny loafers), to first dibs on a wicked pair of lavender suede boots embroidered with a red rose that someone dropped off a year ago and never picked up. The good ones don't always show themselves immediately.

TRADER JOE'S COOKIES
+ A RED TRICYCLE

Amanda and her husband hosted a holiday gathering every year, and when she quit drinking, the raucous, boozy party had to evolve. For Amanda's first year sober, they changed the nighttime event into a "house party" that lasted all afternoon. Amanda knew her guests would expect libations, so she placed a handle of whiskey next to the punch bowl of eggnog. But as guests arrived, Amanda began obsessing that friends who didn't know about her fledgling sobriety were looking for the wine. (More likely, they were enjoying chatting and eating Amanda's cheeseball—her mother's recipe—but Amanda got paranoid about the absence of wine.) Finally she begged a close friend to go buy some wine and beer. Guests stayed and toasted and Amanda felt left out, confused, and, frankly, awful.

The following year, she canceled the party.

But then, in her third year sober, Amanda missed her gathering. She'd had a watershed conversation with Jardine one afternoon, as they drank French-press coffee from Jardine's china cups, a delivery order of Vietnamese sandwiches en route, about how Jardine finally got happy as a sober person when she asked herself what *exactly* she missed from her drinking life, *besides* the booze.

Inspired, Amanda thought about what the *point* of her holiday party had been, what she wanted from it and why. It didn't work to have the party in the same old way and she didn't want to *not* have the party. She loved tradition and an excuse to see people she hadn't seen in a while, to bring new and old friends together. She wanted to celebrate and to be thankful. She hoped her kids would understand their privilege, and wanted to encourage them to seek ways to give to others, especially during the holiday season, which could so easily become a festival of consumption and greed.

Amanda missed that early-party moment, before she drank too much, when she stood in her decorated living room, wearing red or gold (or red *and* gold), all dressed up as she'd been as a kid on Christmas Eve. It was a moment that meant a lot: Amanda had escaped her confusing childhood. She'd made it out, created a family of her own, surrounded herself with kind and wonderful people. Cheers!

So she wanted to replicate that moment without alcohol. It wasn't easy! But perhaps the best things never are. This hard work of sorting out how to make a life sober pays off, because once you discover a new way to host a bash (for example) you don't have to figure it out again. Often the *first* sober anything—the first summer break, or trip, or kiss—is the hardest.

Amanda found a nonprofit center that houses families in need. During the holidays, the organization also gathers wish lists from its residents. Amanda signed up to "sponsor" a few families. She e-mailed friends a party invitation with a link to a spreadsheet if they wanted to donate gifts. She wrote that her holiday gathering would involve tables laden with Trader Joe's cookies and apple cider. She added that guests could bring wine and beer if they wanted to. And then, nervously, she waited.

Amanda's friends showed up with piles of toys, towels, pots and pans, dresses. Sneakers in the requested sizes and wrapping paper and books. Flannel sheets for a single mother. One friend paid a family's rent for the month of December. Other friends brought gift cards to Target, movie theaters, and a PlayStation. Another friend brought a gleaming red tricycle. There was chatting and toasting and platters of chocolates, cookies, olives, and fruit. Amanda can't even remember what people drank, and that's big.

When the party was over, Amanda took a moment in her kitchen, surrounded by gifts and dirty dishes and her kids and her sweet husband, and felt the feeling she'd been missing, but it was even deeper.

The next day, Amanda and her kids delivered the gifts to the organization's office. They toured the housing development and her kids played on the playground with the kids who lived there. When they got in the car to drive home, Amanda's son cried, "Hey!" and pointed out the window. Amanda slowed and they watched a grandmother, mother, and two teen girls coming out of the office building. Riding in front of them was a boy pedaling the red tricycle.

NIGHT-BLOOMING CEREUS
+ WOLF MOONS

Jardine remembers being little and going to a daffodil show at the public library, where all the elder ladies of the small town brought their yellow flowers to be exhibited, with equal parts grace and bloodthirsty competitiveness. It's a memory of variations on a theme: all the flowers were unique, some having tangerine-orange inner cones, others with heavier perfume, one with a bigger collar of pale yellow, another with darker green spears of leaves. There was a sense of ownership from these cultivars, and yet no one can own the workings of a plant, no one can keep it alive when it wants to die, no one can make it appear from nothing. This sense of ephemeral, autonomous life is both frightening and to be celebrated.

Which is the backbone to flower-viewing rituals, like the *hanami* parties thrown in Japan when friends gather to eat and drink under the blossoming cherry or plum trees, reveling in beauty and impermanence. Jardine was at her friend Sunny's place in Brooklyn when the night-blooming cereus in the yard decided to bloom for the first time in fifteen years. This cactus flower is massive, and it goes from a closed cylinder to a giant heady-scented blossom in one night. It gets pollinated by moths and bats during those precious hours when it's open, and then it falls down, it's over, it collapses by morning. So they obsessed and freaked out and watched the whole thing. The bloom was almost animalistic because it happened so fast, opening as they watched, moving in the moonlight, in this Brooklyn backyard. They took a million photographs and grinned like children because it was almost supernatural.

Elegantly dramatic incidents of nature bring people together with a force that feels magnetic. We gather to watch eclipses, dust storms, superblooms, comets. Jardine can even reminisce about going with a posse of early-morning voyeurs to watch two ancient Brooklyn buildings get demolished and blown up. That wasn't nature at work, but it was an occurrence beyond the everyday, and it was bonding, the group standing in the chill of a northern morning, chatting and sipping coffee in the bright light, stranger linked to stranger for an intense moment.

Jardine and her boyfriend were on a patio at a restaurant in LA during a wolf-moon eclipse but were at first focusing more on their grilled Mexican rib eyes than the sky. Sitting at the table to one side, a pair of women talked about something—there was an edge to their conversation, a bitterness. On the other side sprawled a big crew of twentysomething guys and girls, yapping over one another and squealing, superchic and hypercool. Everyone felt separate at their own little tables.

Then suddenly someone stood and pointed, and the whole place looked at the phenomenon in the night sky; they got out of their chairs. Electricity coursed through the circle of strangers. And they shyly, goofily, caught one another's eyes, table to table, like a bunch of middle schoolers at a cafeteria, and all the public-persona armor started to melt away under the red moon.

BROOKLYN BARBERS
+ STRANGERS IN SCOTLAND

The red-and-white-striped pole. The broom that sweeps curls into a dustpan. The way the chair swivels, pumped up or down by the stylist's foot. A mirror handed to you so you can look at the reflection in the wall mirror of the back of your head. To know yourself from a different angle.

That funny moment of paying at the front counter when you feel new and different, and you aren't quite sure yet if that's good, and you smile at the lady behind the desk, and she tells you to take one of the candies in the dish and gives back your credit card and winks and says, "You look fantastic." And even though she probably says that to everyone, you walk into the big city or the small town, and feel a little more like you belong there.

Barbershops and hair salons are intimate spaces. It's not surprising they're the rooms where town gossip is relayed, intergenerational wisdom is traded, and personal problems that are heavy and unrelenting can be laughed at or joked about or maybe just given the light of day so they stop rotting under a rock.

There have been times in our lives when we weren't necessarily friendly to our bodies, but when we went to get our hair done, the act of someone washing our hair and gently scrubbing out the shampoo, then wringing it dry and wrapping it in a towel, brought us back to our senses.

Amanda's longtime hairstylist has helped her adjust to graying hair (she calls the gray streaks "sparkles") and taught her how to wear makeup for a book tour, and even celebrated a wedge of hair she curled forward, calling it a "statement piece." Only in this favorite salon does Amanda let herself preen like a peacock and buy a thirty-dollar lipstick instead of rummaging through the sale lipsticks at Walgreens. Treating herself feels uncomfortable but kind of awesome.

As ladies, we don't get a barber shave every afternoon, but we've always romanticized it: the steam of the towel, the cream, the blade, the rasping noise, the confessions, the inside jokes. When we walk by a busy barbershop for men, we always get a little jealous.

The human touch is powerful. On a grim, dank day in Glasgow (she had tagged along on a friend's work trip but had no work herself), Jardine woke up exceptionally lonely. At some point, she wandered into a department store and a woman coaxed her to the makeup area and said, "Let me do your eyes." Jardine always shied away from this kind of thing, for no reason except that her default setting was to avoid intimate contact with strangers. But she sat on the stool with one boot heel on a rung, tilted her face as directed, and closed her eyes. This woman (whom she didn't know) rested her hand on Jardine's cheek to delicately paint her eyes. They talked about Scotland and they talked about Texas (where Jardine was living), and it was a sweet conversation. Jardine looked in the mirror and grinned because she never would have done these dramatic smoky eyes, but she loved it. The interaction radically altered her mood.

On the completely *opposite* end of grooming and coiffing, there's rebellion against social expectations. "Taking care" can feel like a job—eyelash extensions every three months, fillers here, highlights there, braiding, shaving, painting, waxing, hiding, controlling.

If you've been flattening your hair, why not let it curl and frizz? Dyeing the gray away? Let it glow. Always a clean-shaven man? What about a big, long, streaked beard? Who cares if you get your nails done? Leave them naked for a year to breathe. Do we owe the world a made-up face? Boycott shaving our legs, boycott bras, boycott bathing!

And then one day, throw on some Yves Saint Laurent hot-coral lipstick. Sometimes it feels like we're supposed to choose one ethos and preach it, post it—but screw it. Going back and forth can be fun.

SAGE, EGG SANDWICHES + LOCAL PLUMS

Farmers markets are a banquet for the senses, and a reminder—even for city lushes—of the natural world and its changing seasons. We arrive with cash for coffee and an open mind. We'll wander through piles of figs, zucchini, or fresh avocados, rhubarb, or arugula. Maybe we'll try a hummus or flatbread we've never tasted.

As a local teenager plays guitar at her first gig ever, the prerequisite fedora upturned for coins, we load up on blueberries and raspberries for pancakes; cherries for pies; local jams and jellies; and watermelon just because. The fruits are a riot of color, bursting with flavor. T. S. Eliot asks, "Do I dare to eat a peach?"

The sober lush answers, "Yes."

At the Ridgway Farmers Market in Colorado, there's an Amish family who makes the most scrumptious pies in the world, but you have to get there early or they sell out. The crusts are decorated with birds made of dough. (Amanda invites friends over in the evening, heats up a pie, dons potholders, and brings it outside, pretending—just for a moment—that she could create such divinity.)

Near the pies, Amanda loves to visit with the rescue animals (it's so hard to resist bringing a dog home). She sniffs homemade soaps, feels tomatoes, talks with the elk purveyor, buys fresh sage and a baguette. The goat farmer in a Stetson loves to talk about his cheeses, telling Amanda's daughter about each of his goats. It changes everything to know the stories behind every bite. And always, before settling on a bench or a blanket in the sun, Amanda buys an egg sandwich or breakfast taco that's bursting open with crisp bacon and cheese.

Going to the market doesn't have to mean spending a ton of money—it can be a venture to find one jewel, like a tangerine or blackberry Danish or single peony—to take back home or to work. Or it can be a stroll through the aisles, sampling a paper cup of cider and rubbing basil between your fingers, talking, grazing shoulders with other wanderers. Markets have been centers to town life for a long time, convening us around farmers and artisans and bounty. Feels like we know that walk in our bones.

The funny part is that the first time newly sober Jardine went to a farmers' market early in the morning and saw people buying corn and drinking strong coffee and sitting out in the Texas sun—when the sun was still gentle, before it had heated up midday—she thought, *Who the hell are you?* A secret society of happy citizens she'd never seen. A population of early risers. *Nice to meet you.*

SUPPER CLUBS
+ STAINED GLASS

J ardine used to congregate at a certain bar on a certain night, or at a certain happy hour every Thursday after work, or at a certain friend's house for a certainly rambunctious whiskey-fueled BBQ every other week, and she would know those people were waiting there, and she could count on everyone to revel in the same things (beer! and, to be fair, talking and hanging out and laughing) and she loved having this certainty of certain things and people at certain times.

Is she supposed to replace all that with 12-step meetings? Is that her sole doorway into local community? Is that the only way she can count on a group of human beings who she digs to come together at a regular and recurring time in a fashion that does not need to be engineered by *her*? (Because, ugh, then the success or failure of the "meetup" is on her shoulders and she must organize it and provide potato chips and lemonade . . . Oh no! Anxiety is welling up in her heart as she types. . . .)

Some clubs or meetings will be duds—*it was advertised as a Jane Austen book group, but I'm realizing this is a pyramid scheme*, for example. We think, *My heavens, what did I do wrong to get stuck here? What do I do now?* We could do what Jardine did as a little kid at church: stay put and use the time to look at all the ladies' shoes as they went up for communion and pick out which pair she wanted most. Or we could make up a surreal excuse (*I just got a text that the cat fell into the fish tank!*) and leave, because we're grown-ups and can do what we please. There's of course always honesty as a strategy, announcing that this meeting isn't for us—but that can feel terrifying and we're not trying to feel terrified.

It has been hard to go back and try another unknown after having a few lame experiences, but we've found it essential to keep checking out possibilities. We've found success in just asking around, talking about a desire to explore groups and meetings, and what has turned up is very cool: a supper club a friend hosts at a circuit of homes; a multigenerational women's club that meets monthly to discuss issues that the women present; a fly-fishing group in Pasadena; a group of amateur artists who pitch in to hire a model and do life-drawing classes every other week; a crew of female writers who meet every month or so at a different home and share food and drink and book recommendations.

Whether or not we're religious, we appreciate many aspects of a religious life: the regular convening of friends and neighbors; a reading; a group discussion or contemplation or silence or meditation; the collective energy of singing a song.

While technology can create distance between people, it can also unite us, and there are hundreds of online groups we can join. Amanda has found solace and friendship in an online sober group— it's hard to leave her family at night, and she can check in with her online friends while watching *Queer Eye* snuggled next to her children on her living room couch. Online sober friends are also helpful when we need to vent during a dinner party (we can hide in the bathroom and find support in real time through our phones), in the middle of a tough night (Amanda has texted friends from her closet), or at a wedding where we feel like we're the only sober person in the world (it's possible to have essential company while sitting alone next to a remote lake, crying . . . Amanda knows this from experience).

While we are not recommending anything specifically, we both personally wish we hadn't been intimidated or confused by the prospect of 12-step and other support meetings, and wish we had tried them out sooner. We didn't know it could take time to find the meeting that suits us, as all meetings—and even programs—have a different vibe. We wish we had anticipated the relief of hearing someone say what we thought was our own scary, weird, private truth.

SLOWING DOWN

Making the simple complicated is commonplace;
making the complicated simple,
awesomely simple, that's creativity.

~CHARLES MINGUS

GOLDEN COCKTAIL CART

MILK + ROSES

WILD KINGDOMS

AN ODE TO NOISE-CANCELING HEADPHONES

SEEDLINGS IN THE WINTER SUN

WAKING AT 3:00 A.M.

CHAKRAS

NORWEGIAN TRAINS + POINTY FUCHSIA NAILS

HAMMOCKS

GOLDEN COCKTAIL CART

Once upon a time, Jardine looked at interior design magazines and drooled over the stuff she thought would magically turn her into a grown-up—an umbrella stand, a zebra-print rug, and, of course, the cocktail cart. With its smoked-glass shelves and metal body and perfect little wheels, this piece of furniture would make it official: *You, dear cocktail-cart-owner, are sophisticated and glamorous.*

When you acquire a cocktail cart, you become someone who comes down the stairs in an effortless getup like actors wear when they waltz down steps in classic movies. Casually, as bangles slide up and down your wrist, or a cigar stays put between your teeth, you mix a couple of cocktails and have a witty conversation at the same time, laughing with your head thrown back.

Turns out, at the end of the day, feeling suave wasn't the end-all and be-all. It also turns out that you can decorate the hell out of your space, and you might sit in it and admire your textiles and art and couch and coffee table, and still feel brutally lonely. Jardine had to let go of the dream that owning one specific piece of furniture would make her feel right in the world.

But serving friends *does* in fact make us feel good, like we are connected, and even, sometimes, like we are FANCY. So why not stock a bar cart with an extravagant collection of nonalcoholic ingredients? (Unless, of course, as we want to stress, you might be triggered to drink liquor by dabbling with drink stuff. Companies do make zero-proof bitters, in flavors like plum and Aztec chocolate and lavender, but know that most bitters have a smidge of alcohol to preserve them—so plan accordingly. We've known people on both sides of this decision, and we hope you find your spot too.) The nonalcoholic options these days are increasing exponentially in flavor, concept, elegance, and availability. You can stock jarred tarragon, or quince jam, or wildflower honey. Drinking vinegars, orange-flower or hibiscus water. They make zero-proof aromatic spirits and zero-proof craft cocktails in beautiful bottles, combining ginger and pineapple, or cucumber with juniper and angelica root. Have some chai spice on the cart. Keep a soda maker around for a seltzer base, stock the fridge with herbs or edible flowers or pink rhubarb syrup and coconut water and beet juice, and voilà!

You can collect vintage glasses (emblazoned with a stranger's monogram or metallic iris blossoms) from Goodwill, and add some bougie zebra-print cocktail napkins. The ritual and pomp of making "aperitifs" doesn't have to disappear just because the drinks don't have alcohol. There can still be that slow and easy twilight time with dear friends, when you serve drinks, send around overripe figs and stinky Stilton cheese and walnuts, and watch the sun set lavender and rose, sinking under the horizon.

The cart can also be for yourself, click-clacking the silver stirrer as you concoct some pomegranate-and-ginger elixir on a Sunday evening. Or it can be where you stage the old-school Country-time lemonade and Fritos for the baseball game on TV. You can gruffly pour yourself a Coke with ice from the bucket like a cop from a '70s mystery.

Life is a performance, in the sense that it should be fun, it can be playful, and there are props to consider. We've realized that we'll never stop being set designers to everyday life, but the objects might morph and twist in meaning—something that once stood for an imaginary status, a fictional adulthood, might now signal a very simple hedonism.

MILK + ROSES

We love taking the time for a bath, piling books and magazines on the side of the tub, splurging on bath salts and bubbles. We love Tokyo Milk Eiffel Tower Bubble Bath No. 15; Kneipp's Blood Orange & Black Pepper Bubble Bath; and the bag of Rite Aid lavender Epsom salts Amanda bought in Monteagle, Tennessee, while on a writing retreat. It's this kind of investment in pleasure that we have started to revere. For heaven's sake, we used to spend hours and hours in bars, or at dinner tables drinking—surely we can spend fifteen minutes in the bath?

Indian Ayurvedic practices help us access the idea of bathing as sacred and healing, cleansing body *and* soul. These rituals often start with a self-massage with oil, then proceed to the bath itself—with milk and rose petals or (during cold months) with invigorating mustard and fenugreek. Afterward, we moisturize our skin and dress slowly with care and pleasure. The bath is a time to connect with our flesh, to wake our senses while we relax our muscles.

We can make our own bath salts, if we have the time and inclination. Here's the basic breakdown for a jar of bath magic that will last for months: one cup of sea salt, one cup of Epsom salt, one teaspoon of essential oil (rose, bergamot, eucalyptus—whatever you like!), and herbs or flower buds (a rosemary sprig, hibiscus, marigold petals).

Baths are time for thinking too. Agatha Christie ate apples in the bath and mapped out whole plotlines while luxuriating in warm and sudsy water. Tom Ford and Richard Branson have said lounging in the bath is a key to success. Our favorite bath-hedonist is Liberace, whose marble bathtub had gold fixtures and its own chandelier, in an open marble chamber like a temple—a hallowed place in his Las Vegas mansion.

Liberace knew how to take opulent care of his badass self.

WILD KINGDOMS

When life feels too tame, too orderly, too obvious, too obedient—watch a squirrel ravage a persimmon tree. That's what Jardine is doing as she writes, looking out her window at this tiny beast shaking tree limbs and hunching as it feeds the yellow-orange orb into its teeth, then drops the half-eaten fruit to the patio below. There are plenty of persimmons so the squirrel can be wasteful, and besides, there's no morality in the blue sky of Jardine's backyard. There are just rules governed by fruit and water and leaf and creature.

How quickly the wild things that surround us become invisible as we age! Walking through the South Carolina woods with her four-year-old niece and nephew reminds Jardine of this, because it takes them three hours to cover a tenth of a mile. The kids see everything—a spider web in the abscess of a tree trunk, birds fighting in the treetops, a leaf blighted with something that looks like rust (*What is it? Why is it brown? What happened?* the kids ask), an anthill swarming with ants (*What are they doing? How many are there? How do they get underground?*).

Amanda's kids will only agree to watch one thing together: nature movies narrated by David Attenborough. Sure, the older boys are humoring their little sister as they eat popcorn and watch a film about whales, but everyone's gasps are real when they hear the whale songs.

When we feel jaded or trapped, tuning into animals and insects living on a different plane (but in the same space) can lift us out of human society and human egos. Watching orcas migrate, sitting with a bird-watcher and binoculars and hearing about the species we're seeing, just listening to the coyotes at night, or paying attention for once to the pigeons at our feet in a park in Queens—we allow ourselves to be astounded by their lives, by their hearts beating, by their profoundly different experience on this same planet.

Jardine volunteered at a wildlife refuge center in Texas and nursed orphan wildlife and injured birds and mice. Most of the animals weren't cute and they certainly weren't sweet. They were ugly in their vulnerable states (the baby rabbits were transparent, for example, and rarely survived). It was an education to see how their bodies worked, and to be that close to something *wild*, to think about what that word meant. Bittersweet hours that took her out of her realm.

Animals can connect us to the divine, whatever that means. Watching a beehive operate, it's hard not to sense something beyond our understanding at work. Amanda is learning about birds. Now, when she heads upstairs to sit on her deck after work, she grabs binoculars instead of a glass of Chardonnay. (She still brings a wheel of Brie and crackers.) Tuning into nature's patterns helps Amanda believe in a poetic intelligence that created, and is still creating, her world.

Hummingbirds built their nest in the vines right outside Jardine's kitchen window, so she could see it up close. The nest was tiny, made from repurposed spider web filament, gray and compact. She and Neil watched the eggs hatch, saw the featherless babies getting fed by their mom (a long skinny beak shoved down open tiny beaks), and the babies getting bigger, growing some fluff. But one afternoon Jardine saw the mother bird chirping and flying around the babies in a frantic way. Everything was intact that night before she went to bed. The next morning, the nest was slightly damaged and the babies were gone, and the mother kept flying away, then coming back, hovering, chirping, looking into the nest, hovering more, chirping, looking, frantic. Flying away. Coming back. *Oh no! Was it a hawk? A cat?*

Something had killed them, and the mother had sensed the predator the afternoon before. Who knew this would be so upsetting, so horrible? Jardine cried that morning, feeling like an idiot, like the person who projects human drama onto wild animals, anthropomorphizing them, pinning stuff on their lives they never asked for, all that foolishness. Desperately googling things like *Do hummingbirds mourn? Do animals have emotions? Can young baby birds live out of the nest?*

And then she realized she was ravaging the internet in an attempt to control the sadness by figuring it out and dismantling it. All cried out, red-eyed and chagrined, she finally took her dog for a walk, and the world was electric with sun, the leaves burning emerald, the tiny white flowers on the roadside brambles so bright they were hard to look at. Her own cellular being was lit up with feeling, and this made it possible for her to see the mystery of a vast and complex life cycle in the everyday landscape outside her door, whether she wanted to see it or not. There it was. She knew: *I'm not in charge, I don't understand*, and it was blinding, disconcerting, and beautiful.

AN ODE TO NOISE-CANCELING HEADPHONES

For years Amanda told herself she didn't need the extravagance of expensive noise-canceling headphones. But one of her first sober realizations was that she loved silence. How she had become a grown-up without knowing this (or admitting it) had only one answer: wine. That had been her stillness.

Another revelation she had: She's an introvert. Being around people (other than family . . . and sometimes, OK, even family) for extended lengths of time made her tired, anxious, depleted. But a day alone refreshed her. Maybe *this* was why she drank wine before book-tour events, before parties, during parties. Because big parties and performing in front of lots of people was hard for her.

Once, Amanda said, "I don't want to go to this party, but I need to try to be fun." And her therapist answered, "Reading can be fun."

Reading can be fun! That's crazy talk. Or is it? As a kid, Amanda had known that it was fun, but along the way to adulthood had internalized that staying at home reading was *lame*, the opposite of *being fun*.

Silence became a real priority when Amanda's book deadline coincided with kids home for summer, and she finally looked into noise-canceling headphones. But spending money on herself was *another* thing Amanda didn't know how to do. She bought presents for her children and husband and encouraged friends to treat themselves, but when it came to opening the wallet for herself, she balked. She's proud to wear clothes from college and drive an old, dented car. Whether this is healthy frugality or not valuing herself enough is not always clear.

She bought not one but *three* brands of headphones from Target, test-ran them all, and kept the best one and returned the others. Now, despite the chaos of children with playdates or the roar of an airplane's engines, Amanda can click the blue lever to *on*, and silence fills her ears, washes over and through her like water or mist or light. Silence for many of us is not nothing. It can be everything.

SEEDLINGS
IN THE WINTER SUN

An extremely luscious place to seek out in the dead of winter is a greenhouse or winter garden. We've lounged around in a few over the years, one in Texas full of Meyer lemon trees, another packed with cacti and succulents, and one thick with orchids in the Carolinas. Jardine also visited the Grandes Serres at the Jardin des Plantes, which is a complex of four greenhouses in a botanical garden in Paris. These iron-and-glass structures are right by the Seine, the oldest built in 1635. She went there years ago, and again recently, and each time the same part of her soul woke up the moment she stepped inside.

Maybe it's because the environment is like nothing else—humid, dank with life, hot, and dense with oxygen. The interiors all smell alike to some degree—the fragrance of leaf and soil and sun and water. A place of incubation. Where delicate things can become strong, and beautiful things can bear fruit.

These microclimates are worth tracking down, from conservatories at botanical gardens in London or Virginia to tomato greenhouses in Canada. To be among all that lavish greenery and petal and fruit, to walk through the place and touch a leaf here and stick our nose deep into a bloom—this makes us happy. We can talk or sing to the plants to make *them* happy. We can look at tropical flowers thriving far from home. We can watch frost-tender seedlings get the sun, water, and air they need to grow. We can even bring a sandwich and a book, and sit and read, breathing in that nourishing oxygen, keeping good company with the plants.

Jardine crashed a monthly meeting once of a rare-plants club that was listed in the community section of the paper. A member showed slides of his hiking trip through Mexico and the specimens he photographed along the way. The plants were almost psychedelic in their design, like riddles hiding under boulders and in the shade by a creek. To hear this club talk about how the plants worked and how they were named was extraordinary. Everyone intensely inquired about this or that, occasionally debating a fact, and ate cookies. They asked her name, why she was there, and welcomed her. Jardine didn't know, to be honest, what had led her to the meeting. She was bored, it was there, she was newly sober, and so she went. And she was knocked sideways by the realization that passion is always nearby. We wonder now what we're overlooking, what is surely right in front of us but we can't see it—yet.

Roaming through a hotel or a restaurant, we're never shy about leaning over to sniff the big hot-blood-pink blossom in the vase on the bar. It's a cliché, but we do like to stop and smell the roses.

WAKING AT 3:00 A.M.

(Inspired by the poem "Waking at 3 a.m." by William Stafford)

One great happiness for many new sober lushes is profoundly improved sleep. The deep dreams of a sober person, who was accustomed to waking up throughout the night for years because of too much alcohol and sugar in their bloodstream, are a revelation. And sobriety is in many ways a game of momentum. To wake up one day without a hangover is something. To wake up a few weeks in a row without a single hangover is something else and the momentum builds a conviction that mornings can be good, not awful. To wake up for a few *years* without a hangover establishes an inner trust in sleeping better, and waking up better, and this foundation can subliminally and eventually lead to many things (bigger risk-taking in art or love or business, a general sense of the world's benevolence, more innate faith in our ability to achieve goals, and so on).

It's funny—for Jardine, it was not so much what happened while drinking that made her constantly wonder if she had a problem as much as it was the regularity of terrible sleepless spells in the wee hours. During those windows of time, often from 3:00 a.m. to 5:00

a.m., after a bender or even not-quite-a-bender but still an indulgent night, she was never cognizant enough to talk herself down from irrational anxiety and self-dislike but was also not able to fall back asleep—she was suspended, caught, stuck.

It wasn't moral—she didn't think she was a "bad person" for drinking or doing drugs. The way she acted when drunk at parties wasn't as disturbing as the way she would *feel* in the light of morning when she pulled herself out of a meager shuteye, feeling like death itself. The doom was irrational, the result of a wrecked nervous system, but it was powerful. And she always was forced to realize: *you* made yourself feel bad. Who would do that? She felt vicious disdain toward herself.

But it was unraveling that disdain that led to her retirement from the drinking life. She could not call herself an alcoholic; the word was a barrier, its meaning cobbled together from after-school specials and a limited understanding of addiction. But she *could* understand that it was insane to make herself feel like such absolute shit over and over and over again. Especially when she would often promise to not make herself feel like absolute shit. And then do it again. And then promise. And then do it again. She was finally able to see that this was a disorder of sorts, a dysfunctional relationship with booze, and it wasn't uncommon. And then came the magnificent evolution of cutting herself slack, and giving up trying to control the cycle by just stepping out of the cycle and getting sober.

Amanda had a similar revelation. Her therapist said, "It seems like you can't control your drinking. But once you accept that, and quit drinking, you can stop being mad at yourself for all the times you couldn't control your drinking." *Whoa.*

Not all sober lushes sleep peacefully, but sobriety helps make those can't-sleep-midnight-hours more tolerable. On a weekend getaway, Amanda and her friends laughed at the requirements each had for deep sleep: One friend loved a meditation app. One swore by

"Sleep Stories." Still another needed medication and the sound of thunderstorms.

Amanda is a lifelong insomniac. Even getting sober made no difference: she wakes like clockwork at 3:00 a.m. She's read books about cognitive behavioral training, been in therapy for decades, tried EMDR. She exercises. She's taken kava kava, Benadryl, melatonin, magnesium, GABA, prescription pills, and natural variations of prescription pills. She has a friend in Colorado who makes tinctures and let's just leave it at that. Amanda has an active mind—she's diagnosed herself with *hypervigilance*—it's a problem that hasn't been solved, and so she does her best.

Amanda turns off devices early. She takes medications sometimes, and always mixes up a Calm magnesium drink. She likes to have a hot, rose-scented bath and turn on her essential-oil diffuser. She tucks her sweet little ones into bed, gives her sweet big one a smooch. She keeps a pad and a pen on her bedside table for jotting down things she needs to do or ideas for her novel-in-progress.

Most nights, Amanda tries to run through her day. This is an idea she gleaned in recovery circles: you inventory your day, forgiving yourself for any mistakes, resolving to right wrongs you've made, asking for help, reminding yourself you're not alone. It brings Amanda a great deal of peace.

Getting sober can involve many steps to being more open with oneself, and also letting go of things, and in this way, Amanda learned a lot about managing her brain. When she removed Chardonnay, her brain was raw and sad, needing attention. Every night, Amanda pays attention. Her true heart speaks, and she listens. And then—and she will never not be grateful for this—Amanda sometimes sleeps, and if not, she can be in the dark with herself and feel okay in a new way.

CHAKRAS

We can be hard on ourselves, as if we're two people and one isn't good enough and the other is there to keep mentioning that. We want to be successful at work and love, look great in a bathing suit, be everything for everyone. Or we want to be the proper rebel, follow the ethos of mischief makers, make life gigantic and swanky all the time.

When we stopped drinking, the compartmentalized inner selves—the happy-go-lucky friend, the shark at work, everyone's favorite parent, the lonely misfit—didn't know what to do with one another. We felt like blobs of personality, no longer organized.

Some sleep for a week in early sobriety. Some cry. Some stay in bed for a week eating M&M'S *and* crying. (OK, Amanda.)

Amanda rested for a year or so (see above) and woke up, ready to start being in touch with herself from the root, and tried the 30-Day Yoga Challenge at her local studio. She reveled in the basic act of stretching. Yoga for so many sober people is a way to reconnect with a body, to use that connection as the basis for other parts of ourselves to align and fuse.

And it's a way to "unbend" the body after years of knots and misalignments. Jeez, Jardine used to wake up in horrible configurations, one arm twisted behind the back, eyes glued shut, rigid and fragile like some fossilized skeleton and feeling just as sexy, drool crystalizing on one cheek. Thinking about it now, she imagines all the chakra channels that were supposed to run through her whole self being stopped up, bent, nonfunctioning.

Yoga and Pilates both feel like a gentle, mystical uncoiling of those tubes of energy and light, flooding the self with good vibes. We stay open to new approaches, from sunrise *qigong* at a nearby park to yoga retreats in Thailand with friends we're getting to know.

Watching online yoga instructors is free and can be scheduled anywhere, anytime. For Amanda, an overscheduled cheapskate, this is perfect: all she needs is twenty minutes to hide from her children (with a yoga mat, or even a towel in a pinch) to emerge stronger and calmer. Seeing yoga on the screen and carefully, earnestly, dutifully copying the leader makes us nostalgic for Jane Fonda and primary-color leotards.

Posture—at the core of these practices—is vital to correct the slump that might have come from low morale, typing for hours and hours, fatigue. To walk through the world with head held high is good for us to do even when we don't feel it. Fake it till you make it. And following the breath, focusing on the breath—getting to the marrow of being conscious—maximizes the experiment of sobriety.

NORWEGIAN TRAINS
+ POINTY FUCHSIA NAILS

One of the many simple needs we served by drinking was a desire to space out. To give the poor darling little brain a rest. To mute the ego and all its needy strategizing and surviving and manipulating and narrative-creating. To be calm. To get respite. Especially in the mad world where many of us live—commuting, working, child-raising, dinner cooking, grocery shopping, and bill paying—we all crave an oasis of nothingness.

So add this next idea to the list of things we made brutal relentless fun of, then tried, then loved, then repented for ridiculing: Scandinavian train videos. And ASMR videos like soap cutting and microphone taping. And then there's the crackling-logs-in-a-fireplace videos, and Japanese gift wrapping. And who doesn't love videos of marathon knitting?

Let's start on a platform in a Danish city, the locomotive waiting to set off, and we're watching through the front window of the first car. What exactly are we watching? Tracks leading into an unknown distance, covered in clumps of dirty snow. A whistle—a long electronic beep—the wheels start turning and the engine grumbles and the train moves on these tracks. We rattle through a nihilistic void of a tunnel, *whoosh* out the other side, into the bright light, houses stacked on hills rising from the tracks on each side, now there are more trees, now a body of icy water on the left, fewer houses, soft gray hills in the distance, birds, telephone wires, and now we get it, we're starting to see—this train is going to keep going, and take us with it, with nothing expected of us, no ticket no money no small talk. We won't see anything so astounding that we need to make note. We just ride. For eight hours. And then there's another train getting ready to depart, if we want, through another landscape, for another eight hours. It's like a caravan of abstract deliverance. It unwinds the knots in our mind or soul.

And then—there's slime. And a knife cross-hatching a bar of soap, then shaving off the hexagons of pink, waxy perfection. Brrrrrrr—did you get chills yet? A blond woman who looks like our third-grade teacher but has a Russian accent is using her nails (painted the quintessence of "red") on a white button-down shirt, and we hear the zither of nails on fabric, along with her whispery shared-secret breathless voice that's somehow both there on the TV or laptop but also right here, one inch from our ear, and we can smell the lipstick and feel the heat of her mouth.

We won't go into the science of this effect (mostly because we don't understand it) but we do know that ASMR stands for *autonomous sensory meridian response*. It's about activities that trigger the tingles, as everyone likes to call them, especially on your scalp, for some reason. We think of it as modern spell-casting, and don't need to know why it works to get the shiver, the quiver, the tickle, that helps to calm us.

Atmospheric videos of fireplaces, water lapping on a beach, something stationary but kinetic, repetitiveness being key—these constitute endless internet archives. Slow TV, a concept that comes care of the Scandinavians again, includes the phenomenon of marathon knitting. If you haven't indulged, and you find yourself in a wicked temper one day, please—just check it out. The tactile yarn, the glimmer and click-click of needles, weave on and on and on like a grandfather reading a fairy tale to you, a babysitter braiding your hair, (and unloosing it and braiding it again), until your tiger-soul calms down.

As with all of these online options, from the slime videos to the Swedish trains to the rain and wind and cicadas, there is always the sense that someone made these and put them out in the world. There's a person on the other side of each one. Kind of like the vendors of yesteryear, pushing carts through neighborhoods and hawking fresh-caught eel or shaved ice or coal. Now the handcart is technology, but their wares are just as home-baked and idiosyncratic.

Do we sometimes feel absurd for stoking a fire on our TV instead of in the fireplace? First of all, yes—and that can be the point. It's fun to be absurd. But also—in the confines of an office, in the confines of a stressed-out not-enough-time-for-anything afternoon—a video of bison doing nothing in a meadow somewhere, or boats drifting on a canal in England, or a live webcam of a pond where herons might land any minute but don't, can be a surreal break in the claustrophobic day. Nobody gets hurt. It's harmless. We all need a bit of ambiance sometimes.

HAMMOCKS

L et us make an ode here to napping, to sleeping in the grass, sleeping on a couch, sleeping on a boat or on the beach. Hanging out in a hammock, dozing, dreaming.

It feels sort of wild and unprotected to sleep somewhere besides the bed. Jardine lay dazed in the grass of a public park the other day, taking in the California sunshine, her dog's leash tied to her wrist, and she stared at the big, powdery clouds in the blue sky and the palm tree tops and the jet planes roving through the atmosphere. It felt illicit to be there, to be doing nothing, to be horizontal.

When Amanda and her husband head down to Barton Creek on the hiking trails near their house, they often bring a hammock or two. Hoping for sleep is a stretch, but at least they can relax while their kids play in the cold water.

The hammock is like a physical manifestation of making time in a day—a net slung between trees—a nap carved into the afternoon— a dream given space inside the waking life. The hammock itself could be a logo of defiant pleasure and leisure, the symbol of the nomad, of someone unafraid to just be.

On the Nicoya Peninsula in Costa Rica, Jardine saw surfers from

Israel, from Rotterdam, from Norway, all living in the dense woods close to the beach. They had backpacks, boards, and hammocks, and that was it. And that was all they needed to live for the few months they were here. She also knew a guy who worked in the kitchen of the restaurant where she worked, and he was sick of paying rent, so he had taken to the woods in Texas for a bit. Had a motorcycle and a hammock, and that was it. Smoked his cigarettes after a shift while looking up at the stars, and showered at the YMCA. It didn't last long, but it didn't have to.

There's something, too, about napping—on a beach, on a train, on a friend's couch while they get ready—that reminds Jardine of being a kid, and falling asleep under the table at a dinner party while the parents laughed and ate dessert. We're not in charge. We're sort of lost and sort of found, and someone will definitely, when the time comes, gather us up and take us home and tuck us in. We will be taken care of. Curling up on a sunny October afternoon, with a coat over her, on a friend's rooftop in Brooklyn, sober, and dreamy, Jardine fell asleep for twenty minutes, a half hour at the most, and woke up delightfully confused.

Jardine loves this feeling and might have reached it in the past by drinking enough to be extra vulnerable. It's a weird piece of a drinking life, the way we see people falling apart, uncomposed drunk, and oddly, it can bring us closer: holding a friend's hair back, or comforting a friend who's wasted and bawling. Being wounded, being raw. Sometimes, drunk or high, we would let go of our "image," we allowed people to see us, we were exposed.

Those were real building blocks to real friendships. It's not that napping on a friend's sofa while they make dinner is the same exact thing—but it does create some of the same dynamic. And it's interesting to examine the construction of past relationships, to figure out what brought out tenderness, and to compassionately give it credit—whatever it was—and use it to think about what we want now, and in the future.

CREATING

*An artist paints, dances, draws, writes, designs,
or acts at the expanding edge of consciousness.
We press into the unknown rather than the known.
This makes life lovely and lively.*

~JULIA CAMERON

OH, DARLING, I'M BORED

VETIVER

VIRTUAL REALITY

A WEALTH OF FREE BOOKS

RABBIT HOLE

JAPANESE GLASS PENS

TAKING NOTE

GUERILLA BOUQUETS, IKEBANA + FUNERAL HOMES

OH, DARLING, I'M BORED

Amanda sees it when she takes her young daughter to the beach: with absolutely nothing but sea and sand, Amanda's daughter spends hours building a castle. She invents mermaids who live there. She turns driftwood into boats and shells into furniture. And then, when her castle is washed away, Amanda's daughter runs into the ocean for another hour of daydreaming and jumping in the waves.

Amanda, on the other hand, has at least two novels in her beach bag. The moment her mind wanders, she dips into a book. She has a notebook to make To Do lists. On a sunset walk along the beach, she listens to a podcast. Amanda schedules every moment to be productive. She is utterly terrified of boredom.

At a diner dinner, Amanda's daughter needs only a crayon or two to create art on her placemat, surprising herself (she says) with the images that spring from her mind. Let the adults talk endlessly about the appetizers. Let the other kids kick the table or bend their heads to their iPads. Amanda's daughter understands the power of her own brain.

We try to force ourselves to sustain boredom. This is how great ideas happen! The awful restlessness is fresh ideas and thoughts trying to form, uncomfortably nebulous at first, amorphous. In our early attempts at sobriety, we'd eventually give up after a few weeks or months, saying—in as worldly and jaded a tone as we could conjure—*Oh god, it's just so boring to be healthy. F&*k this.* We were scared of it, lonely, uncertain, and we jumped ship. The sobriety itself was frightening, but we see in hindsight that the boredom was perhaps even more threatening. It's not for the weak. As writers, we know that mental doodling—Amanda draws the three-act structure and imagines ways her novels can play out, or just goes walking and forgets about her manuscript for an hour—allows inspiration to strike. This isn't easy, this patience, this acceptance of suspense, but it's essential. As the writer Gustave Flaubert said, "Be regular and orderly in your life, so that you may be violent and original in your work."

Jardine was at the dry cleaner's, there was a long line, and she was bored, waiting. She was about to check her phone for no reason, to scroll through whatever she touched first, just to be occupied, out of habit, and then she stopped. It was a simple experiment. She looked around—and in the two minutes of simple observation, she noted an old sunbaked calendar on the wall and suddenly jumped back decades to her family's kitchen calendar—Ranger Rick, if her brothers had their way, or the Nature Conservancy. She watched a customer claim a big flouncy flamingo-pink dress—for her daughter's birthday, or prom? Then she sensed something else, and looked over the counter, down to a gray cat hiding under the hanging suits, staring at her. She smiled back at the cat. *I almost missed you, little sweetheart.*

Boredom—our culture treats it like a disease. We must vaccinate against it. Fear it. It's a terrible condition; it means something is wrong. We used to drink for relief from it. We remember chasing away the end of the day, wanting to be sleepy so we could go to bed.

Wanting to be woozy when we got into bed so we didn't have to lie there and think and be stranded with our own selves. But being sober for a number of years has yielded many moments of discovery and new thought, many moments of lying in bed, *not* drunk, *not* sleepy, reading or thinking, and suddenly—a new idea. Or if not an idea, the processing of an emotion instead of burying it in drunken half-sleep. Either way, a moving outward, inch by inch. We haven't exactly come up with a way to live on Mars or an answer to world hunger, but grain by grain, flicker of thought by thought, conscious instant by instant, we're developing paths in our minds and hearts that had previously been untraveled.

Boredom is not just an emptiness for us; it's often the tension of not knowing, not having a narrative, not being entertained. As a culture, many of us desperately ward it off with tablets and TV and pills and cocktails and social media. But that tension is valuable. The price? Discomfort and uncertainty while something brews and grows in the void. The reward? Tiny epiphanies. Daydreams that avalanche into plans. Kittens peeking from under plastic-draped red slacks in a strip-mall dry cleaners in Silver Lake.

VETIVER

t's good to have "moderate" friends—they make our new world go round—our dear partners in crime who drink but never to excess, who abandon a half-filled wineglass when they're done with dinner. (Blasphemy! Insanity! We would NEVER have done that.) They don't understand why and how we sometimes went off the rails, why we had to stop, but they also don't mind and truthfully don't care. Because alcohol just ain't major for them. To them, being fixated on booze is like seeing someone get all hung up on hazelnuts or limes.

Jardine grew up with Alyson Richman, a soulful writer, and a fantastic mate for sober adventures—she's a born moderate who doesn't notice or care if anyone in the room is drinking. So together they devise luscious plans that don't bring them anywhere near booze whenever Jardine is in New York. They scavenge coupons for black-rose facials at the Sisley Spa at the Carlyle. They have sandwiches on the top floor of the Museum of Arts and Design. They also like to dream up creative collaborations and recently went to a perfume designer to make a scent honoring the childhood they shared.

Being writers and innately dramatic, they brought this poor unsuspecting parfumer a rather fanciful and intense account of their childhood worlds, outlined à la Keats-Colette-Proust. She asked what they wanted to evoke with their scent, and they said, *Rhododendrons blooming in pink clusters out of a dark woods. A smokehouse rank with last winter's work. Sand-dusted feet, clamshells, salt-laced air. A boat's teak deck heated by sunshine. And violet shadows moving like snakes on the ground.*

This follows a tradition of poetry between them: Aly and Jardine saw a certain light in each other at the age of *ten*, and immediately set about creating their own secret world drawn from characters in books. They pretended, in Laura Ashley dresses, to be orphans or warriors or dynastic queens.

One summer, when they were twelve, they took pocket Kodak cameras into the woods behind Jardine's house. Taking turns, they posed in kimonos Alyson's father had brought from Japan, a rhododendron behind an ear, lips damp with their first Clinique nude. They dropped the rolls of film at the drugstore, waited with trepidation, and, even though they were rookies, the photographs came out luminous.

How could they lose them! But they did—somewhere between high school and adulthood. Reunited one weekend recently, they talked about memorializing that summer—those pictures—that moment between girlhood and the unknown—without using their usual storytelling medium. They decided to use scent instead.

So they sat at the perfumer's desk, facing shelves of amber bottles filled with the finest grade natural oils and essences as she explained how to build a perfume's "story." How to make the constellation of notes a richer sum than their parts. And they built it step by step, asking, *Can you include rhododendron? How about privet? Is there a way to capture salt, or smoke?* And more abstractly, *Can you capture the thrill of dusk, the terror and beauty of adolescence, the mystery of art itself?*

Once finished, they touched the perfume to pulse points on the wrist and neck, and inhaled. At first, it came on smoky, dense and green, then rushed forward with roses. The rock that stayed was the vetiver, Peru balsam, and a faint whisper of salt from the choya-nak.

Jardine spends more and more time with Aly these days, even though they live on opposite coasts. They talk on the phone for hours and visit when they can. A number of moderate friends have come to the forefront of her life in an organic way, because liquor is irrelevant to them. These were the friends Jardine might have disappointed when she showed up hungover and tired to lunches or movies back in the day. She's glad their friendships lasted through that, and that there's time for a new era and new projects.

VIRTUAL REALITY

We look bizarre from the outside, in padded black headsets, our bodies twisting and flinching as we fly over meadows and cities and woods, enter the dark and psychedelic paradise of Hieronymus Bosch paintings, and swim with whales. We are taking a break from one reality and discovering new ones, with the help of VR.

We touch objects that aren't there, do things we can't do. We fight monsters, we open closets and drawers to solve a crime, we disappear into our own bloodstream. We commit violence. We give birth. We contemplate a Balinese ocean, ride the surf, sleep in the clouds. We zoom into Manhattan or Kauai, pull the sky from dawn to glittering night, and launch our rocket. We walk over a pond of Monet's water lilies and through Marina Ambramović's nightmare of glaciers melting and skies falling. We visit other minds, we fuse our minds with yours, we become strangers, we love strangers, we gain empathy, we are soldiers, we are refugees, we are tigers, we are rabbits, we are lost, we are caught, we are set free.

A WEALTH OF FREE BOOKS

We're both book freaks; we adore the smell of books, the suspense of the narrative, images blooming on pages. Like our childhood heroine, Eloise, we sprawl on our stomachs and read, and worries fade. It's weird that even we, who know that we live for books, can forget there is such companionship and life to be found in them. If we spend time without digging in, some part of us starts to starve and die. Then we remember, step up, and get back into it, and feel lucky all over again.

Amanda worked in a library in college and graduate school, and found solace in shelving books, savoring the yellow light and warmth in the stacks on those freezing Massachusetts (and then Montana) afternoons. She loved the metal cart, its whistling wheels, the way every book had a history—*let's peek at who checked out this account of a group of women who walked from Ouray, Colorado, to Mesa Verde in 1880*—and a place. Amanda volunteers now in her children's elementary school library, putting each book in alphabetical order while the librarian, Tara, reads aloud to the kids in a melodic voice.

The library is a little miracle in any town. It's public, it's free, it's for everyone and anyone, and the purpose of the place is a pure combination of story, information, resources, quietness. *I'll be right there!* Sometimes we just need to get out of the house, out of our own minds. We don't feel like making plans with anyone; we don't want to spend money. We don't need to eat. We don't feel like running. The library opens its arms, and gives us a seat in a big hushed room, opens shelves upon shelves of ideas and stories to us, asking nothing in return. We always feel like we're in good company at a library, hanging with other nerds and curious citizens, not just in the flesh but in the pages and pages and pages around us. If we need a break from the drab monotony of an office job we don't love, we can sneak into the library at lunch, read something transgressive like Clarice Lispector or Xaviera Hollander or look at a Cindy Sherman or Kara Walker monograph, and go back to corporate headquarters, fueled by countercultural vitamins.

Whenever we get that acquisitive itch, and yet we don't really want to pay for it, and we definitely don't want to amass more belongings, a trick is to go to check out a monster stack of library books on vintage cars, gardens, punk-rock posters, architecture, cooking. We pick the biggest, most lavish books they have, and—without dropping a dime—bring our haul home and read for hours, allowing the photos and illustrations to transport us. With a stack of books and a cup of tea, we let beauty wash over us—we don't have to act. No need to *make* the Shanghai soup dumplings from scratch or *visit* Versailles; we don't have to skateboard in a swimming pool or sew the pencil skirt. We can just read about it.

While traveling, we stop in libraries and learn more about the place than any online research could tell us. This is what we used to do by talking up the local bartender, quizzing her on the best hike or café nearby.

To turn this goodness in the other direction, we can stake a "free library" in our yard (or refill a neighbor's library stand), or gather books to donate to the military or to a prison. Amanda attends a party where friends wrap a well-loved book to pass on to another reader. Jardine was once part of a chain where she mailed a used book to someone, and then was on a list to get five books in the mail from strangers. We don't really believe in collecting books as much as circulating them.

We cook with sumptuous books on the counter. We garden with books open on the grass. Our shelves are heavy with old novels and Hollywood biographies and art books and volumes of poems with our mother's name on the front page from when she wrote it there in college. We visit new friends, or they visit us, and we connect instantly by seeing what's on one another's shelves. We don't think we could exist without books.

When Jardine was struggling to finish writing a book years ago, before coworking spaces were a thing, she'd go to the Rose Main Reading Room at the New York Public Library, passing the stone-lion statues that guard the steps, entering into a sacred silence interrupted by a cough or a sigh, settling into the honey of wood and golden light. She was just unable to work at home anymore and needed the strong and silent company, the grand lamps and desks of that space, to keep her going. Writing is solitary but doesn't have to be lonely. Same could be said of life sometimes.

RABBIT HOLE

O h, the magical, glittering, alluring black hole of the internet. How can we say no to you, infinite universe? When we need to say no (through the first half of the workday, for example), we use internet-blocking software so we don't even have to try to resist. The battle is taken out of our hands for a few hours, and this is good because we do *not* have a ton of willpower with this shit.

But that doesn't mean we never explore. And while many studies show we're happier when we turn devices off, it's still a miracle to have at hand what we now have—the internet equals zillions of miles of art and writing and music and ideas and science and video and photography and craft and history. For free. So if we're going down a rabbit hole of online adventures, we might as well be deliberate. We love to think about what will blow our minds and get the creative blood flowing. What will make us feel connected. What will make us feel enlightened. What will make us laugh. What will make us proud of humanity. What will get us high.

That usually doesn't involve fetishizing Lanvin handbags online.

Well, we get sidetracked, but honestly, the more we keep it pure, the better we feel when we snap the machine shut after a couple of hours.

We dig online public-library archives of film where we can watch Charlie Chaplin and his rose, or Maya Deren and the sunlight of her imagination. We love clips of Jack Smith films and abstract video art and interviews with Grace Jones and psychedelic animated short films of dolphins, to trigger new mind states without chemicals. Why not spend an hour of decadent absorption and investigation into kitten videos, French '80s perfume commercials, time-lapse flowers blooming? Or peruse the many websites built by museums around the world, go through the digital hallways of their collections, read about the paintings and sculptures and performance pieces? We listen to music sites' "best of" series, watch all the new videos from trap to punk to pop, write down the names of new bands. We search for quotes on dreaming or horses or heaven.

We keep ourselves, during these periods of luxuriating in the good stuff, from shopping for AAA batteries or athletic socks for a son, even if we need both those things. Because it's a slippery slope from reading an online archive of letters from Martin Luther King Jr. or learning about how Venus flytraps function in the wild to suddenly going into "need" mode, or "buy" mode, or "solve" mode, and leaving the "discover" mode in the dust. We try not to get wrapped up in diagnosing a vague pain we might be feeling (or imagining) in our left forearm. We're not looking to improve ourselves or compare ourselves. Not sinking under a tsunami of despair by poring over the news. Not stalking exes on social media. Not stalking ideas about how we could be thinner or younger or hotter or richer, either. Although the infinite ethernet loves to tempt us in these directions, luring us with clickbait and hyperlinks to worlds made of products and mean girls and bullies and quick fixes. Screw all that.

Stay with NASA's library and watch neutron stars tear one another apart to form a black hole. Stay with footage by a girl who lives on a farm of her goat giving birth. Ransack sites that store the history and sounds of Jamaican reggae. Check out Alison Bechdel's radical cartoons. Read about the 1980 Summer Olympics. Watch BBC clips of a young Alexander McQueen designing a leopard-print dress. Be awed, thrilled, stymied, until your eyes feel sore but your head is buzzing with life.

JAPANESE GLASS PENS

Jardine loves to look through a junk-shop's dresser drawers jammed with postcards of trucks spilling Florida tangerines, or the snow-white pillars of the Parthenon in Athens, or a hand-painted bluebird on a cart of flowers with *Happy Birthday* written in a 1940s font. She picks up postcards, too, when they're paper-clipped to the check at French bistros or offered at art galleries or skate shops; she has one from a religious society that shows a spaceship transporting God. All she has to do is think of someone she misses, write them a little message, stamp and drop it into the mailbox. Doesn't everyone love to get mail? We do; we can't help smiling like a kid when we find a postcard in a stack of bills—a missive from Hawaii where a friend spent their honeymoon, or a photo by Diane Arbus from a sister who just saw an exhibition in New York.

And hotel stationery! We can't ever steal enough. Take the pen and the pad too. It's so exotic these days to write a letter—or to get a letter—and how much better is it when the thing is written on a page pilfered from an old hotel in New Orleans or Morocco?

Modern life is crammed with communications—texts and e-mails and Twitter messages and voicemails. But sometimes the right kind of letter or postcard, a simple thought, an *I love you*, can actually make space in a day, rather than noise. It's something to hold in your hand.

Jardine recently got a glass pen from a Japanese store, and a bottle of murky blue ink called Slumber. These pens were unknown to her, but she was visiting a city where an old friend lives, and he took her to a shop that sells them, knowing she loves to write. It's funny because she was afraid to tell him before meeting up that she doesn't drink anymore, since that's what they used to do together. She thought he'd be disappointed, that there would be nothing to do except make it through a short, awkward dinner. But as often happens, when we give someone a chance, they surprise us. She *did* let him know in an e-mail before meeting that she's off the sauce, and then he came up with this lovely plan, to get a lesson in glass-pen writing from the woman who runs the shop, and then to hit an iconic restaurant next door worth visiting for the people-watching alone. It was a great night, a great reunion, and it yielded a most beautiful souvenir, perfect for writing a thank-you note from the heart.

TAKING NOTE

As writers, we've found that a good tool in sobriety is taking notes on the process. It's a weird thing to be in an experience and also outside it, observing. But sometimes it's soothing—we can reflect on our pain or awkwardness or uncertainty, give it all worth. Whether in a silver-jacketed notebook like the one Amanda bought in Paris or on the back of a Carnival cruise-ship napkin, bearing witness to the world around us is transporting.

It's amazing what we think we know until we sit down to write about it and we uncover some unanticipated piece of the puzzle. We can think ourselves into knots, but externalizing the thoughts can be liberating and really surprising.

"Everything is copy" wrote the glorious Nora Ephron (we miss her so), meaning that she should always see everything happening to her and in her and around her as material for writing and for storytelling. But another layer of this saying is a reminder that no matter how bad things get, we still can tell it as a story one day and hopefully laugh, or at least shake our heads and smile, and whoever is listening can relate or laugh or both.

As Jardine was working on this chapter, she got tangled up in a travel debacle of missed plane connections and was stranded in stormy Dublin, at a hotel filled with football fans coming from the semifinals match. She was pissed at first, too mad to see. But then, after getting cozy in her room, she began writing, and the red haze of resentment lifted from the little horizon of her mind. She wrote about how the hotel carpet was bananas-ugly-psychedelic. Jotted down what her taxi driver told her about cheating at football and understanding mob psychology. The hills outside her window were stunning and wet and emerald green. She realized she was writing this chapter.

GUERILLA BOUQUETS, IKEBANA + FUNERAL HOMES

S upermarket carnations. Giant stalks of gladiolas that almost tip the vase. Oceanfront roses that lose their petals within hours. Buckets of lilacs in the New York rain. Blood-red poppies. Hyacinth heads, with grape-laced perfume. Birds of paradise. Calla lilies. A black tulip, veins of violet and gold. Roadside daisies. One peony.

Flowers have saved our petulant, moody, pessimistic overthinking little souls more times than we can count. Even as a little kid, Jardine constantly fixated on flowers and brought her mother grubby handmade bunches of ancient roses and quince branches and paperwhites. (Of course, it was Jardine's mother's garden that was being ravaged for these bouquets, but the intention was good, Jardine swears it was good, and she stopped when her mom asked her kindly to stop.)

Even though we've never been actresses and never will be, because that has to be the most terrifying job in the world, we love the idea of red roses that fill our dressing room. We love wildflowers that won't last ten minutes in captivity, wilting immediately in the vase. There's a mystique to flowers like lily-of-the-valley that covered the floor of the woods where Jardine grew up, their fragrance leaking into the dark shadows of her childhood, and she has smelled a dozen perfumes that claim to be based on that smell and none of them come close, and she hopes they never do. Flowers are living miracles of art and design, of pollen and stamen and pistil, of leaf and stem.

We read about ikebana, the Japanese practice of formal flower arranging that incorporates concepts of symmetry and counterpoint, and the arrangement is as much a meditative and creative process as it is an outcome. There are flower-arranging workshops everywhere now, and tours through flower markets, and lessons on making plant dye and botanical jewelry.

We love the idea of bringing flowers to a friend for absolutely no reason. We also love the idea of getting flowers and not knowing who they're from. We love spending money we don't have on irises at the grocery store and defiantly walking into the house with them. We steal Queen Anne's lace from the side of the highway and put it in a silver pitcher we found in a cardboard box of "free stuff" outside a house in Los Feliz. We panic before a friend arrives to stay at our house because we think our house isn't good enough and we don't have time or money to go buy flowers—but we realize we can break a branch off the eucalyptus tree outside and stand it in a glass, and it makes the guest room just slightly more beautiful and we feel more like hosts.

It's always a touch of life, of color, of perfume. Whether it's a heavy, dense gardenia reminding us of Marlene Dietrich and a teenage diary we lost and the way cigarettes burn in old movies, or a cedar bough that touches the room with Seattle winter.

Jardine finally got into houseplants too. Up till now she was despondent about her caretaking skills, even for basic plants like philodendrons, with no offense to the philodendron. But a few friends believe plants are a good and simple way to detox homes, and they've been sharing discoveries and tips with her. In particular she's invested in a fiddlehead leaf fig tree despite its reputation for being difficult. That prompted her to go online and find a warren of fiddlehead leaf fig tree worlds populated by fiddlehead leaf fig tree nerds and lovers. They warned that if the plant is yellow near the stem, that means the roots are rotting and that she'd overwatered it without good drainage. If the leaves are brown and crackly at their edges, it's underwatered. She even read somewhere to name her plant, because that strengthens the bond and gives little fiddlehead a fighting chance, and thus his name is Xavier. There are directions about what sun he likes in which months. And she must confess—tuning in to living creatures that share her space, noticing how they're doing, changes how she lives.

There's even something poignant and important about the fetid water poured out after flowers have sat in the vase too long. The stench is incredible, especially because it came from something so recently exquisite. The end is as important as the beginning.

Jardine used to live in Greenpoint, Brooklyn, down the street from a funeral home, and once in a while, she would pick lilies out of its dumpster and take them home. Why shouldn't they have a second life?

ROAMING

There is no end to what can be said about the world.

~JULIA ALVAREZ

BIG-CITY BAD BEHAVIOR—AN ENCORE

ROOM 302

WHAT ABOUT ROME?

DIRT ROADS + PARISIAN BOULEVARDS

FOLLOW ME

AIRPORT ROULETTE

CABIN IN THE WOODS

BIG-CITY BAD
BEHAVIOR–AN ENCORE

Staying up late; talking her way into after-hours bars; having deep, tender, crazy conversations with complete strangers; dancing by herself; forgetting where she was; forgetting everything; breaking the rules of daytime and nighttime and walking into the snowy morning straight out of some party; saying F U to tomorrow . . . Jardine used to love this stuff. Guess what? We still want whatever is at the core of that experience, we still long for it.

It's particularly poignant for her to fly into New York City, which she once upon a time called home, and to see the jewels of light and the topography of cement and brick and tar from the plane, and to get a rush of transgressive memories. This used to be her headquarters for turning life upside down and wreaking havoc on boring conventional expectations.

Her first trips back after surrendering the bottle were hard—she only knew certain pathways through the city, certain rituals, and certain people. She wasn't sure how to even *begin* to do New York City differently. And it felt like being stabbed in the heart with a hatpin—to watch as this glamorous disorder went on around her. But then she realized, after racking up a bunch of phenomenal trips, meeting new people, seeing exhibits, hanging out with old friends but doing different stuff, walking for hours—over bridges and through neighborhoods—that the heart of the city is available to anyone who wants it.

The bottom line is that she *did* sign off on the madness of being blackout-twisted and up till dawn. But she quickly found out that she can *wake up* at dawn instead, cheeks pink with deep sleep, and get a double espresso in Brooklyn and walk over the Williamsburg Bridge in the chilly, misty wind coming off the East River, and meander through the Whitney Museum, looking at mind-bending art. The things she wanted—the sense of anarchy, raw creativity, and connection—could be found at the nightclub but could also be found in the morning, in the exhibition of gold-and-pearls-and-blood Marilyn Minter videos or Hilma af Klint paintings. This rush of empathy or illumination could be located in the early hours as she sipped tea in Tompkins Square and watched characters pass by and wondered about their lives. Beautiful weirdness was hers when she sat at a diner counter in Astoria reading a Mexican comic book someone left on a stoop.

In fact, she started to understand, the anarchy she used to only locate late at night the same way (over and over and over again) had started to feel more like conformity than revolution. And waking up depressed and nauseous after a bender no longer seemed to fit into a breathtaking life. We love you, Manhattan, for taking us as we are, and for always—without fail—giving us a ride. You showed us that there's more than one way into the city's secrets.

ROOM 302

One fact Amanda was never taught in creative writing graduate school is that it's impossible to gaze at your loved ones and be alone at the same time. Sure, they talked about Raymond Carver writing stories in his car, smoking cigarettes and scrawling in a notepad while his children played nearby. But many believe that the serious artist must forgo attachments: the parenting failures of artists are legendary. Amanda sat on a panel next to an incredible writer who, when asked if she had any advice for female writers, responded, "Don't have children."

Then she passed the microphone to Amanda, a mother of three.

Amanda cleared her throat, then spoke the truest words she knows about being a writer and a woman. "Be ambitious," she said. "And when you can, book a motel room."

The tension between motherhood and work was one that Amanda had used Chardonnay to ease. She felt guilty asking for what she needed, which was long periods of time to be alone with her work. To dampen her frustration, she drank. But when that numbing agent was removed, Amanda had to learn to take care of herself, to seek what she needed rather than ignoring it. And so she booked a motel room for one.

There's something so thrilling about leaving your family to check into a motel, the seedier the better. Amanda wishes she could say her writing getaways are chosen for atmosphere, but usually she just books whatever's cheapest on the nights she can sneak off. Though she's dreamed of writing at Austin's Hotel Saint Cecilia or Nantucket's Wauwinet, typing by the pool while someone refreshes her icy lemonade, her personal writing residencies have recently included stays at Gaido's Seaside Inn in Galveston; the Candlewood Suites in Austin; and once, when inspiration struck on her way home from Houston, the Katy Freeway Motel 6.

Amanda's packing list is short: strong coffee, cans of soup, and a box of Triscuits; a warm wrap given to Amanda by an editor years ago when she forgot to bring a coat to New York; a copy of *The Triggering Town* by Richard Hugo; index cards for organizing her plot structure; her laptop; and a folder of scrawled notes, maps, menus, and various research materials. Upon checking in, she changes into her work pajamas and spends a few hours watching TV. There's something so wrong about a working mom watching TV in the middle of the day in a cheap motel that it's got to be right.

As Matthew McConaughey told Amanda, during a late-night Austin City Limits party (who says sober lushes can't have wild nights?), "There's a difference between being alone . . . and being lonely."

In the interest of waking up ready to dive into the work-in-progress, Amanda tries to end her first night watching a movie set in the same place as her novel—Women's Death Row, South Africa, the Texas/Mexico border—or one that reflects themes she's exploring. For her novel *The Nearness of You,* which examines motherhood and surrogacy, she watched the 1988 miniseries *Baby M,* eating crackers and marveling at JoBeth Williams's portrayal of Marybeth

Whitehead clutching her biological child and wailing, "She's my baaaaby!" She can only imagine what her neighbors at the Crowne Plaza on I-35 North thought was going down in Room 302.

And so far, it's never failed. Amanda types for days in complete bliss, and when her motel time has run out, she shows up for school pickup freshly showered and ready to be a mom again. For a while, she makes warm honey milks upon request, spends extra time tucking in each child, does dishes without complaint. Living a dual life has even become a theme in some of her novels as she attempts to suss out what it means to try to have it all, to be a mother and a wife and a writer at the same time. For Amanda, right now, it means remembering to be thankful, being ambitious enough to fight for a motel room of her own, and having a seemingly endless supply of tiny bottles of cheap shampoo.

WHAT ABOUT ROME?

They say you can't travel sober—and, full disclosure, Jardine used to say that too. When she was a drinker, she stated it with worldliness and a jaded half smile: *Oh please, darling, why would you even bother to buy a plane ticket ANYWHERE if you were SOBER!* Now she thinks that's a small-minded way to roam the world. So there's nothing for her in Italy but booze? There's no espresso, no paintings, no gardens of roses, no streets lined with intricate architecture, no *pasta*? And yes, she's gotten *that* lecture from *that* gourmand (everyone has them in their life, or runs into them on a journey), who condescendingly explains that food is "nothing" without wine. She smiles condescendingly back and says, *Thank you for sharing that sweet, dear, provincial little idea of yours.* By now, she's had enough culinary experiences that have demonstrated the massive and magnificent breadth of human imagination to know that there's an infinity to how food is served, to what makes it genius, to how it is shared—and there are no absolutes.

Among the online sober crew Amanda frequents, many members (including Amanda) post that they can handle staying home sober but cling to the dream of drinking on vacation. It's so hard to change the wiring about this, if that's all one has ever known. Part of the luxury of traveling had always meant local drinks, and hours in local bars. Those were the anchors to trip planning. It's especially hard to figure out how to handle a trip if everyone going along will be using these anchors.

We've dealt with this conundrum by remembering that no matter what, here or there or anywhere, sobriety is day by day. You also may not know how you'll feel until you *arrive* on vacation and find you've fretted for naught. Amanda spent time on a cruise ship and was nothing but proud and relieved as she bypassed the eight-dollar glasses of lukewarm white wine and was fully present to enjoy the salty breeze on deck.

Staying sober and allowing all the feelings to cycle through yields quick rewards. And so do hangover-free mornings. We tour Roman ruins, creeping around the vast structures before anyone else is there, just us and the birds in the Italian sky and history. We can do Greenwich Village cheese-shop tours and a walk over the Manhattan Bridge, feeling strong and good (instead of limping along and feeling nauseous and faint and pretending to enjoy it). We camp out in the Colorado wilderness, surrounded by wildflowers, our nights fierce with fire and charred marshmallows, with llamas carrying our goods.

We also conquer some anxiety by front-loading trips with stuff to make us happy and sated and exhausted, instead of just worrying about how to get through long dinners with people drinking wine. We'll skip the tequila tasting in Mexico City, and book a bike tour to Frida Kahlo's house and have a flan after lunch, followed by a nap with the big embroidered curtains of the hotel closed, and then take a swim at a local pool to wake up.

Granted, there are places we've found hard to navigate. Las Vegas is scary with its round-the-clock party in every nook and cranny of the city. All-inclusive beach resorts, where they hand out drinks like free candy, are a constant fear among sober lushes. And events like Burning Man and spring break in Cancun and bachelor parties in Miami and an old friend's grand big birthday held in Ibiza—these all take some strategizing, extra planning, backup-support-solidifying, and midnight phone calls to sober friends back home from restaurant bathroom stalls. When Jardine went to New Orleans, a city she used to imagine as one giant fabulous bar, she laser-focused on the food, hunting down every last sugar-dusted beignet and bowl of crawfish soup, and also the art, and finally the cemeteries, which were quiet and shadowy and thick with star jasmine. It proved to be a perfect trinity, enough hedonism and life and death to satisfy her travel appetite.

Certain locations and events, if they're just too difficult, might be better avoided. We're allowed to choose our destinations.

Then, some places are effortless. Right as she got sober, Jardine was invited by her friend Bradley to Marrakech, where daily life and culinary rituals don't revolve around booze. She took a tagine cooking class in a repurposed almond factory, and the class started late because they were waiting for a fisherman to bring the goods, so everyone talked and talked, and ultimately ate sublimely fresh fish together. She drank sticky rich coffee with rug sellers, and enjoyed a full Moroccan tea service when they hiked into the High Atlas mountains. The server poured steaming water from a brass teapot into glass teacups where stalks and leaves of mint were crushed together with sugar. The African sun dropped behind the wall of the garden where they drank, and all the lostness and disorientation she'd felt during the day swelled up and became awe and pleasure. Traveling sober for Jardine is about making room for "trip loneliness" instead of avoiding it or suppressing it, allowing herself to feel displaced and unsure, and letting all the new and unfamiliar energy of the day mature by dusk, blooming like some kind of night flower into her heart.

You know what we don't miss but thought we would miss so badly it would kill us? The airplane wine in little bottles that costs way too much and meant the person next to us in the aisle seat had to get up eight times so we could pee, and it would also result in the trip starting or ending with a migraine. And it was gross, oaky Chardonnay. Or bland, rancid Merlot.

We worried, too, that getting sober would mean relinquishing the one guaranteed way to meet strangers traveling. Whether it was surfers at a late-night pool in Costa Rica or a couple crossing paths with us in Spain, we used alcohol like a password whispered at the door: *Let's get drunk.* And sure, we made friends that way, allies, heard crazy stories from them, maybe even went on a leg of the journey with them the next day, all of us wounded and bonding over headaches. But we realize now getting wasted together is not the only way to slip dimensions, to find portals, to trip through gates and doors while on the road. We can sit next to people at breakfast in Amalfi, all of us eating ripe apricots and drinking cappuccinos, and ask where they've been so far and where they're going. We can ask backpackers in Prague what they recommend for music, or join a tour of gardens in Kyoto and talk to everyone as we walk, or sit side-by-side with new friends who insist you *have to hear* the magic of Hawaiian slack key guitar.

Travel is psychedelic by nature, as the things we thought we knew or understood melt into a sunset in Kenya or fall like rain in Thailand, and our ideas get turned over and left behind and lost. Travel, if we let it, can make us high on the mineral smell of a lake in Canada or the view from a peak in the Sierras or the human energy coursing through a street in New Delhi. And if we're uncomfortable on a trip, uneasy and out of place, that's usually a sign, we realize, that we'll be changed by whatever we're experiencing and seeing and hearing. We're grateful we no longer erase travel experiences by overdrinking and being hungover. If we did, we wouldn't give these journeys a chance to affect us as deeply, as often, and in such unexpected ways, as they do now.

DIRT ROADS
+ PARISIAN BOULEVARDS

Twilight can be a problem in sobriety, especially at first. We used to mark the line between "work" and "play" with a cocktail, and now we can get irritated and discontent around this "dividing hour" we used to love. We've been jealous when we gaze around a restaurant, watching the boozy calm come over everyone, or when we settle into a deck chair and wish for a glass of something to chill us out on a hot summer evening, or sit cross-legged on a picnic blanket and remember how a drink somehow enhanced everything. We know the bliss was chemical, and we know we can't do it anymore, at least anymore *today*. But we want it all the same.

Here's some sober lush wisdom: when the sun starts to sink, go for a walk.

At her mother's house in Savannah, when Amanda's mother and sisters opened the Chardonnay, Amanda stood and said, "I'm going to have a walk." If her family was surprised, they didn't let on. When Amanda's daughter asked to come along, Amanda held out her hand. At dusk, Savannah was beautiful. A neighbor's cat came to greet Amanda and her daughter. They noticed an azalea bush in wild bloom that they hadn't seen before. They talked and then just strolled. They found their own kind of calmness.

On vacations, aimless walks can take the place of afternoon drinking too. Paris, like many cities that have centuries of history, is a labyrinth of mysterious avenues and doorways. Wandering Edinburgh and San Francisco and Toronto is a pleasure similar to being sober: you don't necessarily have a destination or an answer, you just move moment to moment. You can be lost—not knowing where you're going might be the point.

Amanda does the same walk every morning. She drops her second-grader at school and then makes a slow loop home that takes an hour or so. Not having to think about where she's going allows Amanda to absorb the smells of her neighborhood: rosemary, asphalt, magnolia. She watches seasons change (though in Austin they don't change much). She has an hour to let thoughts rise, to let them leave like storm clouds. This expansiveness makes her calmer all day. Even *knowing* a walk awaits in the morning is a balm.

We *used* to walk to clear our heads of hangover. (Amanda even had a grad-school hike in Missoula, Montana, she called "the hangover loop.") Now it's less a matter of feeling okay and instead it's about walking to feel great, endorphins zinging through our blood, oxygen in our lungs. We can find our way like animals because it's a physical and intuitive activity. Walking costs nothing and can be done alone, or with the company of an audiobook or a podcast, or with a friend.

We read Haruki Murakami's *What I Talk About When I Talk About Running* when we were still drinking, and loved the story of how Murakami started jogging and now competes in marathons. We understood his words "All I do is keep on running in my own cozy, homemade void, my own nostalgic silence. And this is a pretty wonderful thing." But now the passage resonates in a new way.

Murakami writes of just "deciding" to run. He put on old sneakers and exited his home. We can do the same: just open the door and go. We don't have to know how long we'll be gone. It might feel like escaping people or places, but in time, the walk becomes the point.

An unexpected orchard. A horse in someone's barn. A hidden café, a river to cross, a panoramic view from a city's hill. Someone's dinner on the stove puffs out garlicky steam from an apartment window, and a lady waters her roses—we wave, and the lady waves back. Endless possibility instead of one dead end.

FOLLOW ME

Some of us love to run the show. When we're in charge, we don't have to worry about other people making mistakes, or what might happen if our mind . . . *God forbid* . . . has a moment to rest. Heading to Vancouver? We can make a list of restaurants for you. A walk in the park? We'd be glad to tell you where to go and what flowers to look for on the way. We have opinions, plans, direction.

But once in a blue moon, it sure is wonderful to let someone else take over.

One evening on St. Simon's Island, instead of sulking about missing her Chardonnay, Amanda spotted a flier for a half-price kayak tour through the coastal marshes, picked up the phone, and dialed. She showed up the next day with her sister, Sarah, and their children, quelling her own myriad fears (*Were there sharks? What if she paddled the wrong way? Could a kid drown in a shallow marsh?*) by focusing on Sal, a young guide with an impressive knowledge of coastal birds.

Amanda let Sal get her kids into their life jackets. He put the kayaks in the water. "Follow me," said Sal, and all Amanda had to do was agree. As the sun set, they paddled past wrens, egrets, mussels closing up for the night, and even a trio of dolphins, and Sal narrated the story of these creatures for the group. When they were done, Sal helped them pull the boats onto the dock. A handshake, and goodbye—perfect "happy hour" accomplished, thank you!

In Belize, Amanda's boys wanted to do a "waterfall jump" inside a cave. There was absolutely no way Amanda could lead *this* excursion. So they joined a tour and Amanda could be the "cool mom" for making it happen, but she had zero to do with their complicated climbing harnesses or carabiners. (Though she did climb up a waterfall herself, deep inside a cave, and then proceed to freak out, jumping only when the guide explained that her only other choice was climbing back down. Such is life.)

From a Colorado wildflower expedition to a trip to Central America with a naturalist who carried a powerful, heavy telescope to sight a toucan, to a free tour of the Watts Towers in Los Angeles, we relinquish control. We close our eyes. We open them. We hear birds sing. Smell the fractal dimensions of the marsh. Watch the sun set on waterbirds that are watching the sun set on us. If Amanda were in charge, she would have missed so much, caught up in herding and helping and trying hard to answer questions.

It's not just for kids either. On their first day in Hong Kong, Amanda and her husband marched out to find the best noodle shop in the city. They got lost, ending up somewhere that seemed like the right place, but then they couldn't remember—*What were we supposed to order?* Amanda's noodles were odd, fishy. She left defeated.

On their second day, they joined a food tour, and hopping on and off buses at the guide's command, they finally had the chance to talk with other travelers . . . and to each other. They asked what *exactly* was in the bins at the ginseng shop. They tried an egg tart at a historic bakery, enjoyed dim sum in an upstairs hall. They had fun, like kids on a field trip, letting someone else run the show.

Once, Jardine tagged along with Neil to his work conference near San Diego, and she found a free tour of coastal native gardens listed online. The group was led by a native-plant advocate whose weathered face and glittering blue eyes told the story of many years of studying and working by the Pacific Ocean. They looked at dune lupines and sea dahlias, and Jardine learned that nonnative plants don't just struggle to thrive, they also fail to feed the insects and butterflies and birds that have always lived here, and they drain the soil of nutrients and moisture, which contributes to wildfires. She heard lyrical idiosyncratic plant names that held the secrets of centuries of blossoms and leaves and trees and seeds. And they all geeked out over the indisputable power of ecosystems, the genius of their dynamics, and the idea that nothing lives in isolation.

AIRPORT ROULETTE

Back in the day, *airport roulette* meant actually going to the airport on a Friday afternoon and spinning in a circle with closed eyes and stopping to see what gate you're facing, and buying an old-fashioned, carbon-copy paper ticket. Then you got on an airplane to wherever chance was sending you.

Now we like to bring that same gambler's thrill to travel by subscribing to a bunch of flight-deal alerts and fire-sale trip-package newsletters, and by ravaging group coupon sites. Sometimes it's finding a 5-star hotel with a superdiscounted room that *night* in the city next door, since they often offer the rooms that aren't reserved at the last minute, and then you get to spend twenty-four hours out of your regular zone.

Booking a short-notice trip is a way to tell your schedule, *You Don't Own Me*. It's a way to feel like a teenage runaway, slipping out the bedroom window and down the dogwood tree and running through small-town streets to meet your friends. And it's a throw of the dice.

Part of it is risking a dud of a trip, finding yourself and a mate in a lonely little B&B that was half-price for a really good reason. For example, that time Jardine arrived at an Airbnb with eight vanilla Glade plug-ins that made her want to give up on life. And the Craigslist home in Carmel that came with a grizzled homeowner who was convinced Amanda's husband had been sent as a spy and told Amanda and her husband he'd be "just next door keeping an eye on things" for the duration of their formerly romantic getaway.

But then there's this: a retired friend went to China for eight days—plane and hotels and guided tours—for $299. It was the minister of culture of China apparently offering this trip. Our friend went. He didn't just forward the link to friends with *WTF?* written in the e-mail, he didn't just talk about it as we're doing now like a fascinating missed opportunity. He did fast preliminary research to make sure it was legit before the trip sold out, and he went to China. From Los Angeles. For eight days. It was an imperfect trip, and amazing, and it was $299.

We tell a friend to surprise us—we promise we'll pack a bathing suit *and* a ski parka and meet her at the airport. We say yes when someone has an extra train ticket to somewhere we've never considered going before. When Amanda's agent, Michelle, mentioned she'd have an extra bed in her hotel room (and maybe even some writers' conference party invites) in Kauai if Amanda could get herself there, Amanda found a screaming deal and booked the flight. The panic and sheer excitement Amanda felt hitting the Purchase button was worth a million dollars.

Jardine thinks back to the travel-agent offices when she was a kid on Long Island, and tacked to the walls were posters of cherry-red suns and lurid sun-blasted palm trees, tropical oceans and big majestic starfish. Back then there wasn't a mecca of online information about where in the world to go and when, so we asked The Man Behind The Desk, like he was a wizard, who would then point in a direction, and we would go there. We kind of miss that guy.

We've labored over trip planning before and it's paid off. We've also picked up and gone somewhere on a whim, and it's paid off. Even looking at options as they arrive in our inbox, and thinking about packing the suitcases and getting the kids into the car, and then deciding, *Screw it, let's stay home*, can make us happy just to be where we are. But if we can motivate, even at the last second, to go somewhere, to breathe different air, we often come home with a question answered or a tension resolved. Turns out we didn't need to argue about it or figure it out. We just needed to look at it from a different perspective.

When we're feeling down, we get in the car, throw a tent and sleeping bag in the back. We buy pretzels and root beers at the gas station on the corner, and fill the tank. We turn off GPS and drive.

CABIN IN THE WOODS

December 31 was on the horizon. And for Jardine, New Year's Eve has always been *the* holiday, for her whole adult life, that was certified debauchery. Like stay-up-till-noon-the-next-day debauchery. Remember-half-of-it debauchery. Take a week to recover. Trim a few months off her life span. Her first New Year's sober had been the year before, and she'd gone to a huge party, determined to have fun and show the gods of SOCIETY and FUN-NESS who were looking down upon her from the heavens that she still had it in her, that she would not be defeated or slowed down by sobriety.

This year, that didn't feel as necessary, although she fumbled around with options. It had been many, many years of parties. She wondered, *What else is there?*

After much discussion, she and Neil and her beloved cousin Anabel got it into their heads to rent a cabin somewhere pastoral and sumptuous and spend New Year's in front of a fire, watching old movies. Far from everything and everyone. They found a very affordable little house in a town called Tryon, up in the Blue Ridge

Mountains of North Carolina, where cabins are expensive to rent in the high summer season but come cheap in the winter.

It felt odd and disquieting to leave town while everyone else was picking out their violet stockings, their metallic tuxedos, their wigs, their lineup of the night's destinations, their drugs, and their lists of who they wanted to kiss at midnight. Neil and Anabel and Jardine flew to Atlanta with their dog and a bunch of books. Listened to music and podcasts in the rental car, and drove up winding roads, farther and farther from the town below where they bought groceries, till they finally reached a hillside cabin perched so high its windows looked out over all the mountains.

They made a fire, unloaded their stuff, and started chopping vegetables and putting Dutch ovens on the stove and getting dishes going. They'd purposefully picked out food that could cook all day because they thought it would feel good. By the time they ate their stew and bread and beet salad that New Year's Eve night, with dark hills looming around them, stars bright in the sky, the hearth crackling with a steady fire, and they toasted with sparkling apple cider and wished one another good and sweet things in the next year, they all felt like they'd made the right choice in coming here, in choosing this place.

Jardine felt good, too, when she went to sleep, but she couldn't help thinking of what everyone else back in Austin was doing (since, at 1:00 a.m., the night had barely begun), wondering who would go home with who, what the band sounded like, picturing in her mind the glitz and bang of the crowd. She was blissed out and grateful they'd come to the mountains, but part of her still belonged at the party. Had she come to the right place after all? She felt divided, unsure.

It was the next day, when they took a long hike, and the air was so still, they were the only ones hiking in the cold, when she finally understood things. The quiet felt precious. They talked and laughed a lot and the dog ran up and back, sniffing under icy leaves. They shared water and ate apples as they walked, and their faces were pink from that chill. The park was a tiered woods of rhododendron, bushes whose dark moody green leaves were veined with red. She'd grown up with rhododendrons and felt like they were part of a mythology to her life, an elemental plant. She could picture this valley in ecstatic bloom come summertime, the blossoms fat and hot pink and everywhere.

They reached a part of the hike where ancient trees formed a long tunnel, like something from a storybook, and they got to walk under the boughs that connected and laced together above their heads. She could tell by how they were all silent as they passed into this arched channel that Neil and Anabel believed, as she did, that this was a magical space. The hush inside was nothing short of mystical, the stillness like a bell waiting to be rung. She knew her eyes were wet, and she smiled at the same time, because she understood it wasn't at all about finally arriving in the right place, it wouldn't ever be about one right place but always *always* forever exploring.

For anyone reading this who is in need of immediate help with addiction, SAMHSA's National Helpline (also known as the Treatment Referral Routing Service), 1-800-662-HELP (4357) or TTY: 1-800-487-4889, is a confidential, free, 24-hour-a-day, 365-day-a-year information service, in English and Spanish, for individuals and family members facing mental health and/or substance use disorders. This service provides referrals to local treatment facilities, support groups, and community-based organizations. Callers can also order free publications and other information.

There is also a wealth of information online if you search for support meetings in your area.

LAGNIAPPE

AN ECLECTIC APPENDIX OF LUSH RECIPES

Lagniappe is the word used in New Orleans for "a little extra," meaning a gift at the end of a visit, or a tiny delicacy after a long dinner. We hope this collection of formulas and recipes will inspire and delight. We ourselves thrive on luxuriously sober treats as we stumble around the wilderness of daily life, and we also just love the *idea* of them. A rose lemonade fizz (for example) is fabulous when we're thirsty, but the spirit of the recipe itself manages to galvanize us, whether we make it or not.

Included in this chapter are zero-proof drinks (and, as we have noted before, zero-proof drinks are triggering for some of us; please feel free to avoid this section if you find them dangerous); bath milks and bomb formulas; and a medley of recipes from our chapters on movie nights, picnics, bread, honey, bridge parties, and more.

Here's where we raise a glass of coconut horchata to you, wishing you all beautiful things on your own journey, and slip a lavender candy into your pocket for the ride.

DRINKS

THE SOBER LUSH

THE ORCHID THIEF

CHARRED LEMON DRINKS

RED BULL-CRANBERRY MOCKTAIL

ALMOND-FENNEL COOLER

INA GARTEN'S VIRGIN MARY

YUZU, KUMQUAT + CHAMOMILE MOCKTAIL

LAMPLIGHTER INN

JANE'S FONDA'S PROTEIN SMOOTHIE

PINEAPPLE-BASIL SMOOTHIE

MANGO LASSI

HONEYED HOT COCOA

EGGNOG

LEMON, GINGER + LAVENDER
"HOT TODDY"

BATHS

AYURVEDIC HERBAL BATH

BLACK BATH BOMB WITH GLITTER

JAPANESE KOMBU BATH

HOMEMADE LAVENDER OIL

FOOD

HONEY LOLLIPOPS

YOTAM OTTOLENGHI'S FLATBREAD

BRIDGE PARTY PIMIENTO

PICNIC MARINATED SUMMER VEGETABLES

LADY AND THE TRAMP SPAGHETTI AND MEATBALLS

TV-NIGHT TRUFFLE POPCORN

ISABELLE ALLENDE'S *ARROZ CON LECHE,*
OR SPIRITUAL SOLACE

TOLL HOUSE GOURMET CHOCOLATE CHIP COOKIES

DRINKS

THE SOBER LUSH

Jardine worked for years at Justine's Brasserie, a psychedelic, elegant wonderland on the east side of Austin, Texas. She loves dining and hanging out there (Amanda does too!) as much as she loved working there, and the owners, Justine and Pierre, made this drink for her and put it on Justine's drink menu. The recipe was born from their friendship, since Pierre would pick kaffir lime leaves from Jardine's porch tree whenever Justine was cooking a spicy-herby-creamy chicken curry. (Now, the restaurant grows kaffir lime trees in their own backyard garden for savory dishes and to infuse this drink.) Lavender also bridges their worlds because it thrives in the hot springtime fields of Texas as well as in the South of France. But mainly what connects these friends, and what inspired this drink, is the belief that hedonism is for everyone, always, everywhere.

Yields two servings

7 ounces rose-petal tea
Ice
½ ounce kaffir lime syrup
½ ounce kaffir lime shrub
2 drops Le Sirop de Monin Lavender Syrup
Fresh or dried lavender stems, for garnish
Kaffir lime leaves, for garnish
Lime zest, for garnish

1. Make a batch of rose-petal tea, set aside to cool. In a cocktail shaker over ice, add 7 ounces of the prepared tea, ½ ounce of the kaffir lime syrup, ½ ounce kaffir lime shrub, and shake.

2. Pour 4 ounces from the shaker into each martini glass.

3. Add a drop of Le Sirop de Monin Lavender Syrup, and let it sink to make a beautiful purple stripe at the base of each drink; it will be a sweet last sip.

4. Garnish with a sprig of lavender inserted through a kaffir lime leaf, and a sprinkle of lime zest.

KAFFIR LIME SYRUP

1 cup water
1 cup sugar
6 kaffir lime leaves

Bring 1 cup water to a boil. Add 1 cup sugar and whisk into the boiling water. Continue whisking till sugar is dissolved. Remove from heat. Muddle 6 kaffir lime leaves, then add them to the syrup and steep for about 30 minutes as the syrup cools. Use a slotted spoon to remove the leaves from the syrup. Pour the cooled syrup through a fine mesh strainer or multiple layers of cheesecloth into a glass bottle or jar.

KAFFIR LIME SHRUB

Orange peel
6 kaffir lime leaves
1 cup red wine vinegar
2 tablespoons brown sugar

In a jar with a tight-fitting lid, muddle 6 kaffir lime leaves with the orange peel. Add the red wine vinegar. Secure top, then shake vigorously for about 20 seconds, and then allow it to infuse at room temperature for a minimum of 3 days. Add brown sugar and shake again. Once the sugar is dissolved, strain.

THE ORCHID THIEF

We found the recipe for this lovely drink in the New York Times *and we like the idea of wearing silk pajamas while sipping an Orchid Thief, preferably on a rainy evening, playing old records by Lee Wiley and Duke Ellington. Most likely, we'll never quite get around to achieving that trifecta, but the drink can stand for all of it.*

Yields one serving

½ ounce lemon juice
½ ounce orange juice
1 ounce vanilla syrup
Club soda
Orange peel

VANILLA SYRUP
1 vanilla bean
½ quart sugar
½ quart water

1. Slice a vanilla bean lengthwise and add to a quart of simple syrup (equal parts sugar and water by volume). Steep overnight. Remove bean. Store in an airtight container in the refrigerator.

2. Add juices and syrup to a champagne flute. Top with club soda. Garnish with orange peel.

CHARRED LEMON DRINKS

We love seeing the parameters expand for drink recipes, exploding into new ingredients, and even new elements. This drink, from Saveur, *manages to distill the spirit of fire, making a mystical little beverage that evokes volcanoes, sage rituals, and smokehouses.*

Yields four 6-ounce servings

7 lemons, 6 cut in half, 1 cut into wheels
6 limes, 5 cut in half, 1 cut into wheels
½ cup sugar
1½ cups (12 ounces) cold water
Ice, for serving

1. Char lemons and limes: Build a medium-heat fire in a charcoal grill, or heat a gas grill to medium. (Alternatively, heat a cast-iron grill pan over medium-high.) Place 6 halved lemons and 5 halved limes flesh-side-down on grill and cook until lightly charred in spots, 30 to 60 seconds. (At this time, you could also grill the lemon and lime wheels, about 20 seconds per side.) Juice lemons and limes to yield 4 ounces each of charred lemon and charred lime juice.

2. Add the sugar to a medium sauté pan over medium heat and toast, stirring occasionally, until fragrant, 2 to 3 minutes. Let cool for 10 minutes. Add ½ cup of the water, return the pan to medium heat, and stir until the sugar is dissolved. Do not boil or simmer. Set syrup aside to cool; it will keep for months in the refrigerator.

3. In a pitcher, combine the charred lemon juice, charred lime juice, simple syrup, remaining 1 cup water, and ice. Stir until incorporated, and serve in collins glasses over ice. Garnish with lemon and lime wheels.

RED BULL–CRANBERRY MOCKTAIL

This drink, from the Food Lion grocery store chain, is offered in honor of Formula 1 and pinball arcades and motorcycle rides. It pairs well with a hot dog buried under relish and mustard, or fries smothered in hot sauce.

Yields one large pitcher of drinks

1 (12-ounce) can Red Bull Energy Drink

2 cups cranberry juice

1 cup apple cider

2 (12-ounce) cans ginger beer

½ cup fresh cranberries

Lemons, thinly sliced

Ice

Cinnamon sticks (optional)

1. In a large pitcher, place some ice, followed by the Red Bull Energy Drink, cranberry juice, apple cider, and ginger beer. Stir together.

2. In each serving glass, place some ice, a few cranberries, a slice of lemon, and the beverage.

3. Serve with cinnamon sticks, if desired.

ALMOND-FENNEL COOLER

This nuanced and poetic drink is from Jennifer Colliau, a mixologist at San Francisco's Slanted Door restaurant, as published in Food & Wine *magazine. The ingredients list is short and brilliant, the sweet angled perfectly against the citrus, lynchpinned by the anise flavor in the fennel. And come on, who doesn't love a drink with a frond in it?*

Yields one serving

¾ ounce orgeat (almond-flavored syrup)
3 teaspoons fresh lemon juice
Ice
¾ cup (6 ounces) chilled club soda
1 fennel frond, for garnish (optional)

FENNEL SYRUP
1 tablespoon fennel seeds
1 cup water
1 cup granulated sugar

1. In a spice grinder, coarsely grind the fennel seeds. In a small saucepan, combine the ground fennel seeds with water and bring to a boil. Remove from the heat, cover and let stand for 20 minutes. Pour the fennel liquid into a jar through a fine strainer. Add the sugar, cover and shake gently until the sugar is completely dissolved. Refrigerate the fennel syrup for up to 1 month.

2. In a collins glass, combine the orgeat, ¾ ounce of the fennel syrup, and fresh lemon juice and stir well. Add ice, stir in the chilled club soda, and garnish with the fennel frond.

INA GARTEN'S VIRGIN MARY

Ina Garten is so good at purifying things to their essence, and we found her zero-proof Bloody Mary on the Food Network. There are many ways to play on this drink in general, and it helps to start with a good, clean, simple template like this one. Roses are red, and so is tomato juice.

Yields six servings

3 stalks celery from the heart, including leaves, plus extra for serving

2 teaspoons prepared horseradish

1 teaspoon chopped shallot

Dash Worcestershire sauce

1 teaspoon celery salt

1 teaspoon kosher salt

12 dashes hot sauce, or to taste (recommended: Tabasco)

2 limes, juiced

1 (48-ounce) bottle tomato juice (recommended: Sacramento)

1. Cut the celery in large dice, including the leaves, and puree in the bowl of a food processor fitted with the steel blade. Add the horseradish, shallot, Worcestershire sauce, celery salt, kosher salt, Tabasco, and lime juice and process until smooth. Pour the mixture into a large pitcher, add the tomato juice, and stir.

2. Pour into tall glasses and serve each with the top half of a celery stalk.

YUZU, KUMQUAT +
CHAMOMILE MOCKTAIL

Max Reis, the beverage director at West Hollywood's Gracias Madre restaurant, shared this recipe for his yuzu, kumquat, and chamomile tea drink with Good Morning America. *It not only tastes juicy and sumptuous and tangy, the drink looks like a tropical kaleidoscope, or a Carmen Miranda fruit hat, or a work of Mexican paper art.*

Yields one serving

5 kumquats, halved
1 yuzu, halved
1 ounce brewed chamomile tea
1 ounce simple syrup
1 cucumber ribbon
⅓ highball glass soda water
Mint and baby's breath, for garnish

Muddle the kumquats and yuzu in a bar tin. Add the chamomile tea, simple syrup, and a single ice cube to the bar tin and shake vigorously to combine. Fill a highball glass halfway with ice and the cucumber ribbon, and add the soda water. Pour the tin's contents into the prepared glass without straining. Top any remaining space in the glass with soda water and garnish with a straw, mint sprig, and the baby's breath.

LAMPLIGHTER INN

This drink is in honor of the Adult Snow Day, with all its shimmering frosty sleepy luxurious laziness. But it also includes a coffee syrup, so it's a jump-starter, too, when you want to get right into the heart of hedonism and now. *It comes from Alex Jump, the bar manager at Death & Co. in Denver, as published in* Town & Country *magazine.*

Yields one serving

1½ ounces heavy cream
1½ ounces coffee syrup
½ ounce lemon juice
½ ounce egg white
Seltzer
Ice cubes
A couple coffee beans, for garnish

Add all ingredients except the seltzer to a cocktail shaker and shake. Add ice and shake again. Strain into a fizz glass. Top with seltzer and garnish with coffee beans.

COFFEE SYRUP

We like this method (which we found on Nikki G. Davidson's Cocktail Crafty site) because a good coffee syrup can be used in various zero-proof concoctions, or just drizzled on chocolate ice cream or into a yogurt smoothie.

1 cup filtered water
1 cup brown sugar
2 tablespoons ground French roast coffee

Bring water to a boil. Reduce to medium heat. Slowly stir in the brown sugar, and stir until the sugar dissolves. Remove from the heat. Add the coffee grounds to a French press. Slowly pour the syrup over grounds, then stir. Allow to steep for 5 minutes. Slowly press down on the plunger to strain. Pour syrup into a jar or container. Allow to cool before use.

JANE FONDA'S PROTEIN SMOOTHIE

We found this on silverscreensuppers.com, a fabulous archive of movie star's dishes, and the folks at Silver Screen Suppers *pulled the recipe from a video by Jane herself. Jane Fonda is an icon of ever-changing ideas in progress, self-celebration, and hot-pink leotards, and we love her.*

Yields two smoothies

Apple juice (or water) enough to cover the blades of your blender, 1 banana, 2 tablespoons protein powder, 2 tablespoons zero-fat yogurt, 4 frozen peach slices, a big handful of blueberries, and some agave syrup to taste (in the video it looks as though Jane uses about a tablespoon but hard to say). "It's not exactly a science," says Jane.

PINEAPPLE-BASIL SMOOTHIE

This smoothie, by Martha Rose Shulman in the New York Times, *is our ode-to-photosynthesis drink! We love to drink our greens when they taste this herbal and exalted.*

Yields one generous serving

¼ cup tightly packed basil leaves
¼ ripe pineapple, peeled, cored, and cut into chunks (about 6 ounces)

¾ cup plain kefir or yogurt
1 teaspoon honey
1 heaped tablespoon pistachios
½ teaspoon chia seeds
2 or 3 ice cubes

Place all of the ingredients in a blender and blend at high speed for 1 minute, or until smooth. Serve.

MANGO LASSI

We partly love this beverage, from Cooking with Manali, *for its color, the creamy orange-pink of a July sunrise or cheap plastic sandals or a rose in an old painting. The lassi also belongs to the category of drinks that never had alcohol in them, drinks that were created to be just as they are now. Originating in India centuries ago, the lassi can be made with variations of spice and fruit, and is often called the "ancient smoothie."*

Yields two servings

1 cup mango pulp (use fresh if possible from 2 to 3 sweet mangoes, or canned mango pulp)
1 cup plain whole-milk yogurt
½ cup milk (cold), or cold water, to thin out the lassi
1 to 2 tablespoons sugar, or to taste
¼ teaspoon cardamom powder
Pistachios, to garnish (optional)
Saffron strands, to garnish (optional)

Blend the mango pulp in a blender. Add the yogurt and cold milk to thin out the lassi a bit. Also add the sugar and the cardamom powder. Blend everything until well combined. Pour the mango lassi into serving glasses and chill for 20 minutes or more before serving. You may garnish with pistachios and saffron strands.

HONEYED HOT COCOA

Coziness in a glass from Saveur. *Just add a great novel and a roaring fire to achieve winter nirvana. Fair warning: you'll have a chocolate mustache.*

Yields one serving

2 tablespoons honey
2 tablespoons unsweetened cocoa powder
Pinch kosher salt
1 cup milk

Whisk the honey, cocoa powder, and salt in a 1-quart saucepan over medium heat; bring to a simmer and slowly whisk in the milk. Cook, while stirring, until slightly thickened and beginning to bubble at the edges.

EGGNOG

This recipe, by Lacey Baier of A Sweet Pea Chef, *is so light, it will knock you into a dreamy, featherbed-y state of mind! You can moderate the amount of honey per your own desire for sweetness.*

Yields four servings

4 cups unsweetened almond milk
6 egg yolks
⅔ cup raw honey
1 teaspoon ground nutmeg, plus more for topping
1½ teaspoon ground cinnamon, plus more for topping

1 tablespoon whole cloves

1 teaspoon pure vanilla extract

1. In a kitchen blender, add the unsweetened almond milk, egg yolks, raw honey, ground nutmeg, and ground cinnamon, then blend for a minute or so until smooth.

2. Pour the mixture into a saucepan or deep pot, add the whole cloves, and heat over medium heat.

3. Cook the eggnog for 10–15 minutes, until it starts to thicken and slowly cook the eggs. It will be frothy at first.

4. You want the mixture to get hot but not simmer or boil. If it gets close to boiling, you can whisk vigorously and temporarily remove from the heat.

5. Once the eggnog has thickened, turn off the heat and stir in the vanilla extract.

6. Strain the mixture using a fine-mesh strainer to remove the cloves, then pour into an airtight container and place in the fridge to chill for 6–8 hours, or overnight.

7. When ready to serve, we love to sprinkle a little nutmeg and cinnamon on top.

LEMON, GINGER + LAVENDER "HOT TODDY"

From the Kiwi Cook, this is a nice dark-winter-afternoon drink, when you want to get the chill out of your bones, when the sun is gone by 3:00 p.m., when you're sitting by a drafty window at work and have hours to go. This is an electric blanket of a drink, a fail-safe comfort, your own little furnace in a cup.

Serves one (large glass) or two (small ones)

2 cups water

Fresh juice of 1 lemon

2 tablespoons lavender buds

1 teaspoon ginger (or a small peeled knob of fresh ginger)

1 to 2 tablespoons honey or pure maple syrup, to taste

2 green tea bags or 2 tablespoons loose green tea (or choose your favorite herbal tea instead)

1 to 2 crushed (or bruised for a more subtle flavor) raw garlic cloves (optional)

1. Combine the water, lemon juice, lavender, ginger, sweetener, tea, and garlic (if using) in a saucepan. Bring to a boil. Remove from the heat and steep for at least 5 minutes.

2. Strain the brew and pour into a cup or glass. Enjoy warm or cold.

AYURVEDIC HERBAL BATH

This herbal bath, from the Purusha Ayurveda wellness center in Mexico, will help you soak your way to a spicy, aromatic serenity.

3 tablespoons green gram powder

½ tablespoon turmeric powder

¼ teaspoon ginger powder

2 tablespoons rose petals

1 tablespoon raw organic honey

½ cup almond milk or 1 tablespoon almond oil

5 to 7 drops of rose, lavender, or geranium pure essential oil

As you're drawing a warm bath, add ingredients to the water in the order listed. Swish your hand in the water to blend after each addition. Enjoy!

BLACK BATH BOMB WITH GLITTER

A bath bomb to channel the dark energy of late nights and goth parties and tuxedos and cat eyes right into your very own bathtub. Having this little secret waiting at home can make a Vanish even easier, glamorous as slipping into a black limousine. We found this recipe at https://www .steampoweredfamily.com/.

2 cups baking soda

¾ cup citric acid

¼ cup SLSA (sodium laureth sulfate)

¼ cup cream of tartar

1 cup cornstarch

⅓ cup coconut oil

2 tablespoons polysorbate 80

10 to 20 drops each of cardamom and rosemary essential oils

Activated charcoal powder

Black biodegradable cosmetic glitter (optional)

Black decorative sugar

SUPPLIES

Disposable gloves

1 large mixing bowl

Face mask (optional)

1 small microwave-safe measuring cup or bowl

Measuring cups and spoons

Bath bomb molds

Parchment paper

1. Put on your disposable gloves and set out the supplies on a protected table (parchment paper is great for this!).

2. Start out by adding the baking soda, citric acid, SLSA, cream of tartar, and cornstarch to a large bowl. Mix well, but be gentle. Citric

acid can be very irritating if you inhale it. If it bothers you, make sure you work in a well-ventilated space and consider using a face mask.

3. Add the coconut oil to your microwave-safe bowl and melt in the microwave for a few seconds, until it is liquid. Add the polysorbate 80 and your essential oils. Mix well.

4. Add the oil mix to the dry mix and blend everything together.

5. Add in the activated charcoal powder. Remember, this stuff likes to get everywhere! So move gently and slowly. Start by adding 1 table-spoon of activated charcoal to your mix. Once it is blended, if you want it darker, add a bit more.

6. Now you can add in your black glitter if you wish to use it and mix everything together.

7. Use your hands to really mix it in well and make sure there are no clumps or lumps. You will know when the mixture is perfect when it feels like wet sand and you can press the mixture together in your hands and it stays together.

8. If you find the mix is not getting to the wet-sand stage despite exten-sive mixing, it may be that you need a bit more moisture in your mix. If it is dry, just add a little drizzle of coconut oil and mix well until you get the right consistency.

9. Sprinkle a bit of black edible sugar into one of your molds. Carefully add your mixture to both sides of the mold. Make sure they are over-flowing and heaped up; don't pack them tightly, just heap it into the mold sides. Bring the molds together and press firmly. Use a grinding/rotating motion to get rid of the excess mixture. Tap the bomb gently on each end and release.

10. Set on parchment paper and let them sit in a warm, dry area for at least 24 hours. This allows them to harden. Make sure you keep them away from curious hands and curious cats!

11. Once they are hard, store the balls in an airtight container until ready to use.

JAPANESE KOMBU BATH

We found the idea of a kombu soak, kombu being a kelp often used in cooking, in a Tokyo-based online newspaper called Japan Today. *They suggest that bathing in seaweed broth releases amino acids and minerals into the water that are good for your skin. We've also heard that adding sea salt can make the kombu experience even better for your lymphatic system. The savory umami note, found in kombu, is a nice flavor to add to our overall bath rainbow.*

The process is simple. Cut one sheet of dried kombu into 5-cm strips and boil them in a pot of water for a few minutes. Pluck out the kombu strips and add the hot umami water to your bath.

HOMEMADE LAVENDER OIL

We found this bath oil recipe in BBC Gardeners' World Magazine, *and lavender bath oil seems properly English, so the source is ideal. The scent of lavender makes our nerves melt and our hearts open, and while we wish we had a claw-foot tub and broken-down castle and velvet robe and hours and hours to soak and read, we can also be relaxed by simply dabbing oil on our inner wrists.*

Lavender flowers (500g fresh or 6¼ cups/250g dried)
Light olive oil (3 cups/750ml)

SUPPLIES
Small saucepan
Wooden spoon
Coffee filter or muslin bag
Small funnel
Glass container that holds 4 cups, with a wide mouth and lid

1. Gently wash the lavender flowers and leaves under cold, running water, then pat them dry with a paper towel or leave to dry in a colander. Roughly chop them.

2. Put the oil into the saucepan. Heat it gently, but do not allow it to boil. Add the chopped flowers and leaves, stir well, and then leave the mixture to simmer for 3 hours, stirring from time to time.

3. Place a coffee filter into the funnel and use it to strain the oil mixture into a container. Allow the mixture to cool before sealing. This oil will last for up to 1 year if kept in a cool cupboard out of direct light.

HONEY LOLLIPOPS

We found these amber treats by Rita from Design Megillah, who created them as sweets than can be eaten on Rosh Hashanah, the Jewish New Year. We love recipes with history and meaning, candies that carry the hum of a field of wildflowers.

Makes a dozen small or eight large molded lollipops

½ cup sugar
½ cup honey
⅓ cup light corn syrup
2 tablespoons water

SUPPLIES
Lollipop molds
Lollipop sticks
Candy thermometer

1. Prepare candy molds by spraying lightly with cooking spray.

2. In a medium bowl, combine ice and water to create an ice water bath and set aside.

3. Add the sugar to a small saucepan. Carefully pour the honey, corn syrup, and water on top of the sugar, avoiding splashing or dripping on the sides of the pan.

4. Over a medium-low heat, bring the mixture to a boil, stirring gently without splashing, only until sugar dissolves.

5. Boil for about 10 minutes, until a candy thermometer reads 310 degrees. (If not using a candy thermometer, drip a bit of the mixture into the ice water. If it forms a hard candy ball, it is ready. If the ball is still soft, cook a few moments longer and repeat.)

6. Remove the pan from the heat and immerse the bottom of the pan in the ice water bath for about 20 seconds to stop the cooking. Carefully wipe dry all water from the pan before proceeding.

7. Pour the syrup into the candy molds. Add the lollipop sticks and twist the stick so that the tip is coated in syrup.

8. Allow to cool and harden at room temperature. The lollipops should be hard, shiny, and ready to pop out of the molds and wrap in plastic in about 15 minutes.

9. Store the lollipops wrapped individually in plastic (bags or wrap) at room temperature in a well-padded, airtight container or freezer-weight ziplock bag for up to 7 days. The objective is to keep air and humidity from making the candy sticky.

YOTAM OTTOLENGHI'S FLATBREAD

Ottolenghi is a journeyperson in the culinary arts who we like to emulate. He's quoted in The Guardian *(where we also found his recipe for flatbread) as saying: "I don't like people telling me what to eat and I don't like to tell people what to eat." This is such a beautiful kind of hospitality, to offer something without forcing it.*

Yields eight servings

1 teaspoon fast-acting dried yeast

6 ounces warm water

1 teaspoon caster sugar

½ cup plain natural yogurt

2 cups plain flour, plus extra for dusting

2 cups strong bread flour

1 teaspoon kosher salt

8 tablespoons ghee, for frying

1. Whisk the yeast, water, and sugar in a small bowl, set aside for 15 minutes, until it starts to froth, then tip into an electric mixer with a dough hook. Add the yogurt, flours, and salt, and knead slowly for 2 minutes, to combine; the dough will be quite dry. Turn up the speed to medium-high and knead for 5 minutes, until the dough is smooth yet firm. Roll into a sausage and cut into eight pieces. Roll each piece into a ball, put on a large tray, cover with a clean tea towel, and set aside to double in size (about 90 minutes).

2. Roll each ball, one at a time, on a lightly floured surface into a 7½-inch-wide circle. Melt 1 tablespoon of ghee in a nonstick frying pan over medium-high heat, and fry the bread for 3 to 4 minutes, turning halfway, until golden brown on both sides. Set aside, cover with a clean tea towel, and repeat with the remaining dough and ghee.

BRIDGE PARTY PIMIENTO

A parlor-room sandwich in honor of Amanda's grandmother's bridge parties, adapted from a recipe by Natalie Chanin and Butch Anthony and discovered in Bon Appétit. *Perfect with a ginger beer.*

Yields eight servings

1 red bell pepper
1 jalapeño
¾ cup mayonnaise
1½ teaspoons Worcestershire sauce
¼ teaspoon cayenne pepper
⅛ teaspoon paprika
1 pound sharp cheddar, grated
Kosher salt and freshly ground black pepper
1 ciabatta loaf, halved lengthwise, lightly toasted
Pickle slices (for serving)

1. Roast the bell pepper and jalapeño over a gas flame, turning often, until the skin is blistered and charred all over, 5 to 10 minutes. (Alternatively, broil on a rimmed baking sheet.) Transfer to a medium bowl and cover with plastic wrap; let steam 10 minutes. Peel and seed the peppers, then finely chop them.

2. In a medium bowl, mix the mayonnaise, Worcestershire sauce, cayenne, and paprika. Fold in the cheddar and chopped peppers; season with salt and black pepper. Spread on the ciabatta and slice crosswise into pieces. Serve with pickles.

DO AHEAD
Pimiento cheese can be made 5 days ahead. Cover and chill.

PICNIC MARINATED SUMMER VEGETABLES

Tuck these chilled vegetables into your basket on a sunny day, as per Bon Appétit.

Yields six servings

3 summer squash or zucchini (about 1 pound), sliced on a diagonal
½ inch thick
3 red, orange, or yellow bell peppers, cut into 1-inch strips
4 tablespoons extra-virgin olive oil, divided
Kosher salt and freshly ground pepper
2 garlic cloves
2 tablespoons sherry or red wine vinegar
4 sprigs oregano

1. Place racks in upper and lower thirds of oven; preheat to 475 degrees F. Place the squash and bell peppers on separate baking sheets. Drizzle each sheet of vegetables with ½ tablespoon oil, season with salt and pepper, and toss to coat. Spread out in a single layer, turning the peppers skin side up.

2. Roast the peppers on the upper rack and the squash on the lower rack, turning squash once, until tender, 15 to 20 minutes. Let cool slightly; remove the skins from peppers.

3. Whisk the garlic, vinegar, and remaining 3 tablespoons oil in a large bowl; season with salt and pepper. Add the vegetables and oregano; toss to coat. Cover and let sit at least 1 hour.

Vegetables can be made 3 days ahead. Cover and chill; bring to room temperature before serving.

LADY AND THE TRAMP
SPAGHETTI AND MEATBALLS

We love the idea of a movie night with friends, where the pressure is off and the food is comforting. When showing Lady and the Tramp, *what better meal than spaghetti and meatballs, from feastofstarlight.com?*

Yields two servings

MEATBALLS

- ½ pound ground beef
- ½ teaspoon kosher salt
- ½ teaspoon freshly ground black pepper
- 1 shallot, minced
- 1 garlic clove, minced
- 1 teaspoon dried oregano
- 1 teaspoon dried thyme
- ½ teaspoon red pepper flakes
- 1 egg yolk
- ⅓ cup bread crumbs
- ¼ cup buttermilk
- 2 tablespoons grated Parmesan cheese
- 1 tablespoon canola oil

TOMATO SAUCE

- 6 ounces dried spaghetti pasta
- 2 tablespoons olive oil

2 garlic cloves, minced

2 shallots, minced

14 ounces DiNapoli crushed tomatoes

Salt and freshly ground black pepper, to taste

Fresh basil leaves

Grated Parmesan, to taste

1. To make the meatballs: Combine all the meatball ingredients except the canola oil in a medium bowl. Mix together with your hands and gently form them into balls, approximately 1½ inches in diameter. Be careful not to press the meat together too tightly. Place the meatballs in the refrigerator for 15 minutes. Heat a large skillet over medium heat with the oil. Once it is hot, add your meatballs in batches so they have space around them. Cook until golden brown on all sides. Repeat this step for the rest of the meatballs. Set aside and save the pan for the sauce.

2. Meanwhile, bring a large pot of water to a boil with 1 to 2 tablespoons salt. Once it comes to a boil, add your pasta and cook until al dente.

3. Make the sauce: Heat the same pan you used for the meatballs over medium heat and add the olive oil. Add the garlic and minced shallots and cook for 2 minutes, until soft. Add the crushed tomatoes and scrape off any of the bits left over from the meatballs. Simmer the sauce for 10 minutes. Add the meatballs and simmer for another 5 minutes. Season with salt and pepper.

4. Once your pasta is cooked to al dente, strain and transfer the pasta to the pan. Toss it in with the sauce. Add in the torn basil and serve immediately with basil to garnish and freshly grated Parmesan.

TV-NIGHT TRUFFLE POPCORN

Amanda loves to cozy in with her family to watch movies (or Queer Eye, *or nature shows) and eat popcorn. Chef Graham Elliot featured this recipe at the Food & Wine Classic in Aspen, during a demo called American Classics 2.0.*

Yields two servings

½ cup popcorn kernels
1½ tablespoons corn oil, for stovetop popping (optional)
1½ tablespoons unsalted butter, melted
1 tablespoon truffle oil
1 ounce Parmesan cheese, finely grated with a microplane (about
   ¼ cup)
2 tablespoons chopped fresh chives
2 teaspoons salt
1 teaspoon freshly ground black pepper

1. Pop the kernels in a standard hot-air popper or in a covered deep saucepan with corn oil.

2. Transfer the warm popcorn to a large bowl, and add the butter and truffle oil. Toss well to coat the popcorn.

3. Add the Parmesan, chives, salt, and pepper. Toss well.

4. Transfer the popcorn to a brown paper bag or a serving bowl. Serve immediately.

ISABELLE ALLENDE'S
ARROZ CON LECHE,
OR SPIRITUAL SOLACE

Our sensual inspiration, Isabelle Allende, suggests covering your lover from head-to-toe with this indulgent pudding and licking it off. When you're finished reading her glorious "Memoir of the Senses" Aphrodite, where we found this recipe, you may just be in the mood. And there's always the option of savoring this warm treat on your own.

Yields eight servings

½ cup rice

4 cups warm water

10 cups milk

1 cinnamon stick

2 cups sugar

1 piece lemon zest

1 tablespoon cinnamon

Soak the rice in warm water for 30 minutes. Drain. Cook the rice as instructed on package, with the milk and cinnamon stick until the rice begins to soften, about 30 minutes. Add the sugar and lemon zest, and simmer over very low heat, stirring from time to time to prevent the rice from sticking. In about 30 minutes the mixture will thicken. Place in a bowl, cool in the refrigerator, and sprinkle with the cinnamon just before serving.

TOLL HOUSE GOURMET CHOCOLATE CHIP COOKIES

Amanda's top-secret recipe . . . don't forget to use a bit of extra brown sugar and Mexican vanilla!

Yields twenty-four servings

2¼ cups all-purpose flour
1 teaspoon baking soda
1 teaspoon kosher salt
1 cup (2 sticks) unsalted butter, softened
¾ cup granulated sugar
¾ cup packed brown sugar (plus a bit extra!)
1 teaspoon vanilla extract (Mexican is best!)
2 large eggs
2 cups (12-ounce package) Nestlé® Toll House Semi-Sweet
    Chocolate Morsels
1 cup chopped nuts (any kind)

1. Preheat the oven to 375 degrees F.

2. Combine the flour, baking soda, and salt in small bowl. Beat the butter, granulated sugar, brown sugar, and vanilla extract in large mixing bowl until creamy. Add the eggs, one at a time, beating well after each addition. Gradually beat in the flour mixture. Stir in the morsels and nuts. Drop by rounded tablespoon onto ungreased baking sheets.

3. Bake for 9 to 11 minutes or until golden brown. Or a bit less, if you like them gooey, as Amanda does. Cool on baking sheets for 2 minutes; remove to wire racks to cool completely.

4. Eat them hot.

ACKNOWLEDGMENTS

We would like to thank the two women who supported the idea of *The Sober Lush* from the start—our agents and friends Michelle Tessler and Sally Wofford-Girand—and our fearless editor, Sara Carder. We are thankful for the whole team at TarcherPerigee, including Rachel Ayotte, Anne Kosmoski, Lindsay Gordon, Sara Johnson, Megan Newman, and Allyssa Fortunato.

Amanda would also like to thank her beloved family: Tip, Ash, Harrison, and Nora, as well as her sisters, Sarah Ward McKay and Liza Bennigson, her brother, Brendan Westley, and her beautiful mother and dashing father-in-law, Mary-Anne and Peter Westley.

Jardine dearly thanks all her beloveds who read this early on, who taught her lessons about a lush life, or who inspired her to think differently! Neil, Cari, Bradley, John, Chris, Johnny, Aly, Arielle, Debbie, Johnny, MC, Justine, Denise, and Pierre.

We also thank the many friends and strangers who have shared their stories and ideas with us over the years.

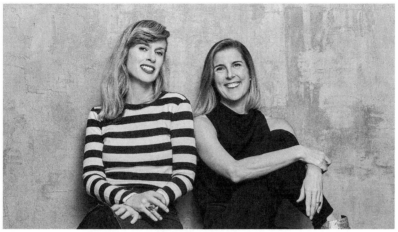

Jardine Libaire is the author of the novels *Here Kitty Kitty* and *White Fur*, and she currently lives in Los Angeles.

Amanda Eyre Ward is the author of seven novels and a collection of short stories. Her work has been optioned for film and television and published in fifteen countries. She lives with her family in Austin, Texas, and Ouray, Colorado. Her newest novel is *The Jetsetters*.